KT-501-014

Telephone Consultations in Primary Care

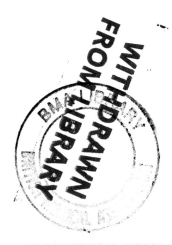

WITHDRAWN FROM LIBRARY

BMA LIBRARY

BRITISH MEDICAL ASSOCIATION

0790344

Telephone Consultations in Primary Care

A practical guide

Tony Males

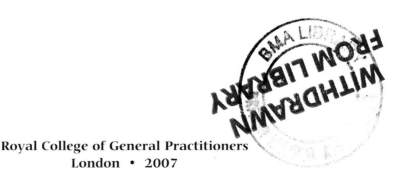

WITHDRAWN FROM LIBRARY
BMA LIBRARY

Royal College of General Practitioners
London • 2007

The Royal College of General Practitioners was founded in 1952 with this object:
'To encourage, foster and maintain the highest possible standards in general practice and for that purpose to take or join with others in taking steps consistent with the charitable nature of that object which may assist towards the same.'

Among its responsibilities under its Royal Charter the College is entitled to:
'Diffuse information on all matters affecting general practice and issue such publications as may assist the object of the College.'

British Library Cataloguing-in-Publication Data
A catalogue record for this book is available from the British Library

© Royal College of General Practitioners 2007
Published by the Royal College of General Practitioners 2007
14 Princes Gate, Hyde Park, London SW7 1PU

All rights reserved. No part of this publication may be reproduced, stored in a retrieval system, or transmitted, in any form or by any means, electronic, mechanical, photocopying, recording or otherwise without the prior permission of the Royal College of General Practitioners.

Disclaimer
This publication is intended for the use of medical practitioners in the UK and not for patients. The authors, editors and publisher have taken care to ensure that the information contained in this book is correct to the best of their knowledge, at the time of publication. Whilst efforts have been made to ensure the accuracy of the information presented, particularly that related to the prescription of drugs, the authors, editors and publisher cannot accept liability for information that is subsequently shown to be wrong. Readers are advised to check that the information, especially that related to drug usage, complies with information contained in the *British National Formulary*, or equivalent, or manufacturers' datasheets, and that it complies with the latest legislation and standards of practice.

Designed and typeset by Robert Updegraff
Printed by Hobbs the Printers Ltd
Indexed by Carol Ball

ISBN: 978-0-85084-306-4

Contents

About the author

Tony Males is the senior partner of a city practice in Cambridge, one of six partners in a paper-light, purpose-built surgery operating the Advanced Access system alongside nurse telephone triage. He developed his interest in telephone consultation through the now disbanded Fenland Research Group and focused on the out-of-hours aspects of doctor communication through this medium in his MSc dissertation in 2000.

Tony is also employed part-time by the University of Cambridge in the General Practice Education Group, sharing responsibility for the development and delivery of the undergraduate primary care curriculum. Tony contributes to the practice-based teaching of Cambridge medical students and is a trainer. He was successfully nominated a Fellow of the Royal College of General Practitioners in 2004.

Tony is married to Becky, also a GP, and they have three children.

Introduction

The telephone is both a blessing and a curse to health professionals. With it they can attempt to distinguish the minor illness from the potentially serious condition, follow the progress of patients with chronic disease or who are making difficult lifestyle changes, and provide information about treatments and investigations. The clinician is at the mercy of anyone capable of using a telephone; patients and their carers can summon medical help from almost any location, at any hour, whatever the weather and at little expense.

Guidance for general practitioners on conducting out-of-hours telephone consultations and home visits was published before the introduction of the 1990 General Medical Services (GMS) contract.[1] The following decade saw rapid changes in the expectations of patients and the delivery of primary care services. Crouch et al.[2] (London, UK) identified factors external to the National Health Service (increasing use of telephones and help lines in popular culture and demand for healthcare services, particularly out-of-hours) and needs within it (to manage limited resources, improve access and quality of care, find new methods to deliver out-of-hours services and extend the roles of nurses) that have led to a growing interest in the use of the telephone in clinical care. The authors conclude: 'Telephone advice may offer a means of managing waiting times and appointment systems more effectively through providing patients with readily accessible assessment and self care advice, and prioritising their need for medical attention.' Within the targets of the 2002 NHS plan[3] and the obligations of the 2004 GMS contract[4] lies the fulfilment of these earlier predictions.

Telephone communication

Telephone dialogue is context-dependent and can vary from informal interaction between close friends, which resembles everyday speech, to formal exchanges between professional and client, buyer and seller, employer and employee, which sound like actors reading from a script. When our telephone rings we bring to the call our current thoughts, feelings and activities from which we have been interrupted, incorporating some into the conversation. When we make a telephone call we prepare what we wish to say to a greater or lesser extent and modify our agenda according to the verbal and non-verbal feedback from the person at the other end of the line. In medical telephone calls each party behaves according to certain institutional and social rules, the same rules that govern the face-to-face consultation and enable patients to reveal personal details about their lives and bodies, and give permission for health professionals to use their knowledge and skills to serve patients, transcending the usual social and physical boundaries.

Benefits and risks

Requests for appointments, repeat prescriptions, referrals, laboratory and medical imaging results can all be handled by telephone in primary care, but the fundamental unit of medical care, the consultation, is the most common and most written-about use of the telephone in medicine. Patients, their carers and clinicians exchange the costs and inconvenience of a face-to-face appointment for the cheaper, quicker yet riskier medium of the telephone when consulting at a distance. A common symptom such as headache has such a far-ranging differential diagnosis that assessment by telephone history alone is beset with medico-legal pitfalls.[5]

Health professionals are trained in the art of observation, drawing data from their patients as they walk, talk and move when dressed, and from the appearance and feel of their uncovered bodies. The elimination of these traditional sources of information leaves the clinician in a relatively cueless environment, relying on improvisation and common sense as he or she attempts to apply the theories of communication and the experience gained in clinical work to problems presented through speech and non-speech sounds while trying to practise safely – both for the patient's sake and in defence of his or her medico-legal position.

Telephone technology

The guidance in this book is based on the telephone as essentially an audio device. Videophones are now available and are likely to become commonplace; whether their use in medicine affords an advantage by providing valuable visual cues remains to be established. The use of the telephone is expanding in other ways. Technological advances have enabled data other than speech to be transmitted along telephone wires and through wireless signals: fax messages for handing over clinical problems from one service to another; mobile telephone text messages for reminding patients about their appointments; ECGs in order to help a cardiologist diagnose an arrhythmia; and photographs of skin lesions for the dermatologist to offer an opinion. Contemporary primary care is telephone- and information technology-dependent; practices and out-of-hours service providers are able to improve the access to and quality of clinical care for their patient population, and to network more effectively with the local health economy, by exploiting the potential in a well-designed telecommunication system.

Intended readership

This book is intended for GPs, GP registrars, foundation-year doctors in general practice, practice nurses and nurse practitioners, practice receptionists, out-of-hours service call handlers and paramedics. The multi-professional environment of primary care requires a common set of skills, including the ability to communicate within and between professional groups. It is not only the patient who consults in primary care: nurses also consult doctors and vice versa, paramedics may seek advice from the scene of an emergency, and GPs often call upon their consultant colleagues as an alternative to referral. The telephone is ideally suited to these examples of inter-professional communication.

Aims of the book

The aims of this book are: to guide primary care professionals in the appropriate use of the telephone when speaking with patients, carers and colleagues; to raise awareness of the limitations of telephone communication; and to improve the accuracy of triage, diagnosis and advice-giving. Guidance in these areas can be found at the end of each chapter in the form of boxes of bullet points for easy reference.

Health professionals and their support staff receive training in their face-to-face communication skills but these may not be sufficient to prepare them for the unique medium provided by the telephone.[6] Therefore readers are encouraged to take an active role in their professional development in this area by attempting the exercises in each chapter. Transcripts of telephone consultations appear in several chapters and have been reproduced verbatim except for the names of places, patients and doctors, which have been changed to preserve anonymity. Consent to use the transcripts for publication and training purposes was obtained from the parties concerned and with the approval of the Cambridgeshire Local Research Ethics Committee.

Overview of chapters

The ten chapters are grouped into three parts: the principles of telephone consultation in primary care; telephone consultations and the primary care team; and clinical management by telephone. Chapter 1 is a summary of telephone use in medicine in recent decades and Chapter 2 explains the differences between telephone and face-to-face communication. The third chapter covers the limitations of telephone consultation and the mixed success of training for health professionals. Chapter 4 considers the ethical issues of consent and confidentiality as well as the risks, benefits and resource implications of telephone consulting. The next three chapters describe telephone communication in general practice during normal working hours and out-of-hours between callers and administrative staff, nurses (including the use of decision-support software) and GPs respectively. Some inter-professional communication issues appear in these chapters but Chapter 8 explores them in more detail. Chapter 9 takes 15 common presentations that can be assessed and sometimes managed by telephone advice alone, with reference to published guidelines. The final chapter looks to the future of remote consultation through media other than the traditional landline.

Acknowledgements

I am grateful to Cambridge City Primary Care Trust for providing prolonged study leave funding, to my partners and staff at York Street Medical Practice and colleagues at the Department of Public Health and Primary Care for releasing me from my duties for a year, to my locums for covering the work and to my family for allowing me to use our sabbatical for writing. Rodger Charlton and Helen Farrelly at RCGP Publishing have been most encouraging during the whole process and the help of Julie Draper, Julian Cooper and Maureen Duff has been invaluable.

References

1. Knox JDE. *On-Call: Out-of-hours telephone calls and home visits*. Oxford: Oxford University Press, 1989.
2. Crouch R, Dale J, Patel A, Williams S and Woodley H. *Ringing the Changes: Developing, piloting and evaluating a telephone advice system in accident & emergency and general practice settings*. London: Department of General Practice and Primary Care, King's College School of Medicine and Dentistry, 1996.
3. Department of Health. *The NHS Plan*. London: Department of Health, 2002.
4. The NHS Confederation. *Investing in General Practice: The new General Medical Services Contract*. London: The NHS Confederation, 2003.
5. Kavanagh S. Diagnosing acute headache: avoiding pitfalls – a guide to practice. *Medical Protection Society UK Casebook*. London: Medical Protection Society, 2003, pp. 8–14.
6. Reisman A and Brown K. Preventing communication errors in telephone medicine. *Journal of General Internal Medicine* 2005;**20**:959–63.

PART 1

The principles of telephone consultation in primary care

CHAPTER 1

The history of telephone use in primary care

The telephone was invented by Alexander Graham Bell in 1876. Three years later it had been successfully exploited in family medicine:

> The Yankees are rapidly finding out the benefits of the telephone. A newly made grandmamma, we are told, was recently awakened by the bell at midnight, and told by her inexperienced daughter, 'Baby has the croup. What shall I do with it?' Grandmamma replied she would call the family doctor, and would be there in a minute. Grandmamma woke the doctor, and told him the terrible news. He in turn asked to be put in telephonic communication with the anxious mamma. 'Lift the child to the telephone, and let me hear it cough,' he commands. The child is lifted, and it coughs. 'That's not the croup,' he declares, and declines to leave his house on such small matters. He advises grandmamma also to stay in bed; and, all anxiety quieted, the trio settle down for the night [reproduced with kind permission of *The Lancet*].[1]

The accumulated literature over the subsequent 130 years made one editorial writer feel as if the main function of the telephone 'was to keep patients at arm's length'[2] while another welcomed the relocation of the access point for health care from the surgery into the patient's sitting room.[3] This chapter covers the progress made in the primary care telephone management of patients and carers over the past 40 years, first the work pertaining to daytime practice, then to the out-of-hours period. Figure 1.1 summarises these developments in the context of primary care evolution in the UK. For a comprehensive history of British general practice the reader is referred to a text edited by Loudon, Horder and Webster.[4]

Telephone use in office hours

GPs in the United Kingdom have been slow to take advantage of the telephone compared with family physicians in the United States.[5] Hallam's comprehensive review of the international literature cites work from several US sources.[6] Owing to the lack of a convention for classifying medical telephone calls it was not possible to make comparisons between studies but telephone consultations accounted for at least 15

Figure 1.1: The development of telephone use in primary care

Telephone consultations constitute 25% of doctor–patient contacts in the USA	7% of doctor–patient contacts via telephone in UK	Access to UK GPs via telephone limited despite patients' willingness to consult via this medium	Trials demonstrate cost-effectiveness of telephone triage and telephone-mediated management	Nurses more involved in chronic disease and minor illness management by telephone

Office hours   Workload increasing, primary care teams expanding   New appointment systems introduced

Out-of-hours   Increasing use of rotas and deputising services   Development of GP cooperatives

39% of GPs on call five or more nights per week	7% of GPs on call five or more nights per week	Wide variation in percentage of calls managed without face-to-face contact: 5–74%	Similar variation in telephone advice rates in cooperatives Nurse triage in cooperatives shown to be safe, effective and to reduce GP workload

Night visit fee introduced   GPs begin to employ practice nurses   GMS contract revised   NHS Direct established   New GMS Contract   Organisations run out-of-hours service   Primary Care

1960   1970   1980   1990   2000

per cent of doctor–patient contacts, up to 45 per cent in paediatric practice, and an overall average of 25 per cent in the USA in the 1960s and early 1970s. There were roughly equal numbers of clinical and administrative calls. Calls about children were more likely to result in a subsequent face-to-face consultation and patients from higher socio-economic groups used the telephone for consulting twice as frequently as those from lower groups. Despite the greater use of the telephone in medicine in the USA, it is rare for doctors to charge for patient-initiated telephone consultations.[7]

Access to daytime primary care by telephone

Between 1978 and 1985 the number of UK households with a telephone increased from 67 per cent to 81 per cent but the percentage of office-hours doctor–patient encounters that took place by telephone remained the same during this period at 7 per cent.[8] In 1981 the Acheson Committee expressed concern over telephone access to GPs in London.[9] In order to address this the authors of a King's Fund Project investigated the literature relevant to London general practice.[10] Despite the national trend in telephone ownership, the proportion of poor families and elderly people with domestic telephones was low. Public telephones were more likely to be out of order in the more deprived areas. British Telecommunications was also criticised for not making available appropriate technology, such as call diverters. For patients who did have access to a telephone, the systems for taking messages, transferring and answering calls were confusing. Allsop and May described the telephone communication situation in London in the early 1980s as 'haphazard, undocumented and subject to the idiosyncrasies of individual practitioners'. They recommended codes of practice, research and education in telephone consultation.[10]

Even by the end of the 1980s telephone access to GPs in the UK was still limited. Two thousand GPs were surveyed in 1988 of whom 1459 (73 per cent) responded. Of the respondents 848 estimated receiving four or fewer calls from patients per day. The ratio of registered patients to incoming practice telephone lines was 3659:1.[11] Hallam recommended that this ratio should be 2500:1.[12] In a survey of patients reported in the same year, 67 per cent thought they should be able to talk directly to the doctor by telephone but 61 per cent had never tried.[13] Patients rated this service more highly than better receptionists, longer surgery hours, longer consultations, shorter response times to requests for emergency visits, and improvements in surgery premises. Hallam echoes the recommendations of the King's Fund Project in her 1992 paper on access,[14] suggesting that practices should publicise telephone access facilities, document the consultations and develop guidelines on the management of problems suitable for telephone advice. By the turn of the 21st century a Dutch practice was overwhelmed with requests for telephone consultations: a mean of 165 calls during the special telephone hour that the doctors had made available for patients.[15] The introduction of an assistant trained in reception and some medical tasks to triage the incoming calls enabled the GPs to gain control of their workload once again. This process of organisational change reflects the conflict between controlling access to primary care health professionals and providing personal, continuing care. In an interview study conducted recently in the northwest of England, GPs, practice nurses and practice managers acknowledged this tension but justified triage in the context of demand management and the evolving roles of the members of the primary healthcare team.[16]

The use of the telephone as an administrative tool

Although triage aims to sort patients according to biomedical diagnosis and allocate them to appropriate management, the telephone has been put to other uses in order to improve access and clinical outcomes. Higher rates of influenza,[17,18] pneumoccocal[19] and pre-school[20] vaccination have been achieved through telephone reminders compared with letters. Telephone prompts also help to improve patients' attendance rates, such as adolescents at a hospital clinic[21] and adults at a community mental health clinic.[22] Glycaemic control, self-care and symptoms improved when diabetic patients were telephoned every two weeks for a year[23] compared with a control group of diabetics receiving usual care. The intervention included a series of computer-generated telephone messages and questions, to which patients responded by using their keypads, as well as human contact by a nurse. Of 400 patients receiving a prescription after a face-to-face consultation in rural Sweden, those randomised to a follow-up telephone call a week later to remind them to have the medicines dispensed were more likely to do so.[24] Interestingly female patients were more likely to respond to the prompt than male patients, whose rate of prescription redemption was lower in both the control and intervention groups.

The role of nurses in daytime telephone consulting

Nurses and nurse practitioners in primary care have played an important role in the development of telephone use, especially with the introduction of NHS Direct, which will be covered in the next section of this chapter (p. 13). The routine management and follow-up of several chronic diseases lend themselves to protocol-driven nursing care. An example of research in this area that involves the telephone is provided by a trial conducted in four practices by members of the General Practice Airways Group.[25] Two hundred and seventy-eight adult patients were randomised either to be telephoned to have their asthma reviewed or invited to attend a face-to-face review with a practice nurse. In the intervention arm 74 per cent of patients were reviewed compared with 48 per cent in the control group. Quality of life scores and clinical indicators were similar in the two groups. The study was criticised for its low rate of recruitment of eligible patients and concern was raised over the lack of peak expiratory flow rate measurements and examination of inhaler technique afforded by telephone review alone. A trial comparing usual care with additional telephone contact by primary care nurses for the management of depression was reported from California (USA).[26,27] It showed significant improvement in the Hamilton Depression Rating Scale and Beck Depression Inventory scores as a result of the additional ten telephone calls during the first four months of the augmented group's antidepressant treatment. Another US study demonstrated improvement in clinical outcomes for depression when telephone follow-up was included in a resource-intensive quality improvement trial.[28]

Primary care nurses also manage minor illnesses,[29] and conduct triage and give advice via the telephone.[30] These papers refer to single practice teams who documented respectively the process of training an existing practice nurse to undertake face-to-face minor illness consultations, and the effect of nurse telephone triage on GP workload. Gallagher's research (Tyneside, UK) claimed a 54 per cent reduction in doctor workload although he acknowledged that the study period included the quieter summer months.[30] Eighty-eight per cent of patients who responded to a postal questionnaire (response rate 71 per cent) were satisfied with the service. Three randomised controlled trials were reported in the *British Medical Journal* in 2000[31–33] demonstrating equal clinical outcomes from, and greater patient satisfaction with, nurse consultations compared with doctor consultations for minor illnesses. Nurses conduct longer consultations than GPs and give more information about minor ill-nesses and their self-management. With nurse telephone triage[34] patients are more than twice as likely to receive telephone advice only and almost four times as likely to be managed by a nurse in a subsequent face-to-face consultation compared with GP same-day appointments with no available triage system, but even at the turn of the 21st century triage systems in daytime primary care were uncommon.[35]

The role of GPs in daytime telephone consulting

A team from a 14,000-patient practice in Bolton (UK) set up a dedicated telephone advice line.[36] Most of the 277 calls taken in the five-month study period in 1989 lasted around three minutes. If the advice line had not been available 75 per cent of patients who responded to the follow-up questionnaire (response rate 55 per cent) said they would have made an appointment for a face-to-face consultation and 13 per cent said they would have requested a home visit. Ninety-one per cent of respondents were satisfied with the advice line and the doctors in the practice thought that 64 per cent of the calls were useful. A New Hampshire (USA) group substituted doctor-initiated telephone follow-up calls for face-to-face consulta-tions in a primary care setting between 1988 and 1990.[37] Five hundred middle-aged and elderly male veterans were randomised to receive three telephone contacts and a doubling of their usual face-to-face consultation interval, or usual care. Over the course of two years the telephone care patients used significantly fewer prescribed drugs and experienced fewer admissions (and those who were admitted had shorter hospital stays) resulting in savings of $1656 per patient. There was no significant difference in mortality between the two groups.

In the more recent past a team of physicians made themselves available for tele-phone consultations in New York (USA) for three weeks and saved around 60 emer-gency room visits.[38] McKinstry and colleagues conducted a randomised controlled trial of GP telephone triage in two practices in West Lothian (UK) to examine the effect of the intervention on GP workload and quality of care.[39] Although four and three-quarters hours of doctors' time was saved during the four weeks of the study, patients randomised for triage and managed by telephone alone were more likely to consult again in the subsequent fortnight, reducing the impact of this workload reduction. This study was criticised for being small[40] and for not distinguishing between telephone consultations conducted for triage purposes and those for com-plete management.[41] Jiwa was more optimistic in his team's paper from Sheffield (UK).[42] The saving was a 40 per cent reduction in demand for same-day face-to-face consultations but the cost was a 26 per cent increase in the practice's telephone bill.

Telephone use out-of-hours

Out-of-hours primary care has evolved alongside increasing patient demand, both the rising number of out-of-hours calls and the heavier workload during office hours. Less personal commitment and continuity of care, and greater use of on-call rotas, deputising services and cooperatives, led GPs to question the continuing need for and sustainability of 24-hour responsibility and availability. Hallam's 1994 literature review[43] covers the period from the 1960s onwards. In addition to rising demand, financial incentives may have affected doctors' decisions whether or not to visit patients out-of-hours, but the introduction of the night visit fee in 1967 enabled national data to be collected. In that year the number of night visits per 1000 population was 4.3. This figure rose to 10.1 in 1976,[44] to 15.5 in 1981[45] and to between 14 and 35 in the period 1985–9.[46–49] Thirty-nine per cent of GPs were on call five or more nights per week in 1964 compared with 9 per cent in 1977. The average number of hours on duty in 1989–90 was 26 per week, the equivalent of a one-in-four rota.

GPs' responses to out-of-hours telephone calls

There is considerable variation in GPs' responses to out-of-hours calls, even in the same locality.[50] GP trainees Cubitt and Tobias described out-of-hours calls in two London (UK) practices covering about 24,000 patients during four consecutive weeks in 1978.[51] The differences between the framing of presenting problems and the visiting pattern of the doctors seemed to relate to differences in the organisation, culture and personalities involved in the practices, which were otherwise identical in terms of patient demographics. One practice, described by the authors as 'paternalistic' because of the directive nature of the doctors' interactions with patients, gave telephone advice to 31 per cent of callers, while the other, called 'democratic' for its collaborative approach, advised 49 per cent. Marsh and colleagues wrote up a year's worth of data collected by two out of five partners' calls in his Stockton-on-Tees (UK) practice.[52] An unexpected 59 per cent of calls were managed by telephone advice in the year 1984–5, which generated considerable debate through the subsequent correspondence. The highest rate published was 74 per cent in a rural practice.[53] A 24 per cent telephone advice rate was reported by Livingstone from two years' data from two East London (UK) practices[47] and a mean of 37 per cent (range 5–57) in a survey of 13 practices in North London (UK) by McCarthy and Bollam, also from the mid-1980s.[54] Most of the practices in this survey used deputising services for part of the out-of-hours period. Practices with a low telephone advice rate used deputising services more than those with a high telephone advice rate. Deputies were far more likely to visit patients when called compared with the GP principals who employed them, partly because there was no alternative location available to them and partly for financial reasons as the night visit fee subsidised the charge made by the deputising service.

GP cooperatives

General practice cooperatives began to develop in the late 1980s. The expansion of this method of managing demand and improving the duty doctor's quality of life was facilitated by changes in GPs' terms of service allowing the doctor on duty to judge whether and where an out-of-hours consultation should take place,[55] and the provision of the Out of Hours Development Fund by the Department of Health.[56] There is just as much variation in the proportion of calls managed by telephone alone in the context of a GP cooperative: 10 per cent to 65 per cent (median 38 per cent) reported by the 67 respondents to a postal questionnaire sent to 98 UK cooperatives in 1996.[57] A comparison was made by Salisbury between the services provided by a deputising service and a GP cooperative in London (UK) in September and October 1995.[58] The former took 1810 calls and gave telephone advice to 365 patients and carers (20 per cent) while the latter took 3798 calls and advised 2267 (60 per cent). A sample of patients was sent questionnaires to determine the level of satisfaction with either the deputising service or the cooperative. The questionnaire was a slightly modified version of the instrument designed and validated by McKinley et al.[59] The response rate was 67 per cent and, unlike earlier surveys indicating high levels of satisfaction with nurse-led telephone triage and minor illness advice during office hours, patients were less satisfied with telephone advice by doctors out-of-hours. Patient dissatisfaction with telephone consultation was a theme found in a systematic review of the various types of out-of-hours services available in the UK.[60]

The out-of-hours system in Denmark underwent reform in 1992 with the introduction of county-based services replacing GP rotas and deputising services.[61] Patients' out-of-hours telephone calls were answered and triaged by GPs, fewer of whom were required to run the service. In a study based in one county[62] the proportion of out-of-hours contacts managed by telephone alone rose from 22 per cent to 50 per cent and the home visit rate reduced from 57 per cent to 21 per cent. After the change, 71.3 per cent of patients were satisfied or partly satisfied compared with 87.3 per cent in 1991, the difference attributed to the greater use of the telephone. These data reflected the national picture.[63]

The role of nurses in out-of-hours primary care

Out-of-hours services then developed to include nursing colleagues in telephone consultations. In the mid-1990s the South Wiltshire Out of Hours Project (SWOOP) Group (UK) demonstrated the feasibility,[64] safety and effectiveness[65] of experienced practice nurses working in GP cooperatives using the decision-support software Telephone Advice System (TAS © The Plain Software Company). In a randomised controlled trial the nurses managed 50 per cent of the 7148 calls in the intervention arm by telephone and without referral to a duty doctor. This is a similar result to the nurse-led triage service for paediatricians in Denver (USA),[66] which also met with the satisfaction of parents and doctors alike. NHS Direct was introduced in 1998 by the Labour government that had come into power the preceding year.[67] Staffed by nurses 24 hours a day, this service was intended to complement existing primary and secondary care services, and improve access to information and services either by telephone or via the internet. It began in three pilot sites in England (Lancashire, Milton Keynes and Northumbria) and became a nationwide

facility in 2000. Publicity was in the form of local press coverage, local radio adver-
tisements and house-to-house distribution of leaflets.[68] NHS Direct had its sceptics[69]
and protagonists.[70] On the one hand it seemed to encourage contact by the 'worried
well' but on the other it appropriately diverted as many callers towards self-management who would otherwise have contacted a GP or attended casualty departments as it did from tentative telephone enquiry to urgent or emergency care. It
received 68,500 calls in its first year from a population of 1.3 million, of which
72 per cent were out-of-hours. The study from which these statistics were taken[71]
demonstrated no difference in patients' use of accident and emergency (A&E) or
ambulance services, and a small but significant 3 per cent decrease in the use of GP
cooperatives in the pilot areas. A postal survey was also conducted in the early
days of NHS Direct[72] of 1050 callers, 719 of whom (68.5 per cent) completed questionnaires. Ninety-five per cent of respondents thought the advice they received by
telephone helpful and the outcomes were as follows:

- 1 per cent were diverted to an emergency service
- 21 per cent of callers were advised to attend A&E
- 20 per cent were advised to consult a GP immediately
- 25 per cent were advised to consult routinely
- 26 per cent were advised about self-treatment
- 7 per cent were advised to contact another service.

Nurse-led telephone triage systems exist in other countries such as Sweden,[73]
Canada[74] and the USA. Data were reported on over 8000 calls to a paediatric after-
hours call centre in Philadelphia (USA), representing activity in four separate
months in 2000.[75] Eighteen per cent of parents were advised to take their children
to the emergency department, 27 per cent to arrange contact with a paediatrician
within 24 hours and 41 per cent were given advice on home treatment. The state
of Western Australia introduced the country's first nurse-led telephone triage service in 1999[76] initially in urban and suburban areas, and then to the rural population. In a nation with such a low population density outside the main cities, telephone connections are a vital means of accessing health care. Examples of telephone-based services for palliative care patients and their carers[77] and for people
experiencing psychiatric symptoms[78] in remote rural areas have been reported in
the Australian literature.

Recent developments

An independent review of English out-of-hours services published in 2000[79] advocated national quality standards in the areas of access for patients, specifically the
requirement for care to be provided through a single patient- or carer-initiated telephone call, and integration with other out-of-hours services, in particular NHS Direct.
Services were required to meet the standards by November 2002. The contributors
recommended that GPs be given the contractual option of delegating out-of-hours

clinical responsibility to appropriate services but it wasn't until April 2004 that the new General Medical Services (GMS) Contract[80] for GPs became operational. The 2004 GMS contract between GP practices and Primary Care Organisations (PCOs) allowed practices to opt out of their 24-hour responsibility. PCOs are the NHS bodies responsible for providing primary care services in a practice's locality through employing health professionals and contracting services to GPs, dentists, pharmacists and opticians (Primary Care Trusts in England and Wales, Health and Social Services Trusts in Northern Ireland and Health Boards in Scotland). In October 2004, PCOs took over the responsibility for providing out-of-hours services to their populations, typically around 100,000 people, either by managing a service themselves, commissioning it from an accredited provider, or by monitoring the quality of a service provided or secured by individual practices. These latter two options may prove to be suitable for the remote rural areas of Scotland and Wales. A new framework for the introduction of standards in the NHS as a whole was introduced in 2004 with both a patient and public health perspective.[81] Out-of-hours service providers were requested to comply with the National Quality Requirements by 1 January 2005.[82] Features of the Requirements relevant to the telephone consultation are:

- no more than 0.1 per cent of callers will find the line engaged
- no more than 5 per cent of incoming calls must be abandoned (an abandoned call is defined as one where the caller discontinues the call after 30 seconds, allowing time to listen to a message that may be played before the call is answered)
- all calls must be answered within 30 seconds, or within 60 seconds of the end of an introductory message
- immediate life-threatening conditions must be identified and passed to the ambulance service within three minutes
- clinical assessment of urgent calls must be initiated within 20 minutes
- clinical assessment of all other calls must be initiated within 60 minutes
- after clinical assessment the patient must understand what is to happen next, and when.

Practical application

Primary care teams have been learning about the advantages of the telephone and experimenting with its many applications over the past few decades. The adoption of US telephone consulting practice is slow but not necessarily appropriate in the UK context. The service provided by primary care in the NHS is free at the point of delivery whether face-to-face or by telephone. GPs still offer home visits – a rarity across the Atlantic – and the population density is higher here hence neither doctors nor patients have far to travel. There is an opportunity cost in introducing telephone triage, advice and follow-up: practice nurses and nurse practitioners are taken away from their other clinical tasks and need time to gain the additional knowledge and

---

Box 1.1 Guidance on telephone use in primary care

- Practice teams should regard the telephone as a means of improving access and personal care rather than as a barrier.

- Patients should be involved in any plans to develop or change the telephone-based services a practice provides.

- A practice should have one incoming telephone line per 2500 registered patients and the flexibility to open further lines at times of high call volume.

- Out-of-hours service providers should have sufficient incoming lines to meet the National Quality Requirements.

- All incoming and outgoing telephone calls with patients and carers should be documented in the medical records.

- Reception and call handling staff should be trained and deployed to respond efficiently to incoming calls, including the initial triage of clinical and administrative calls to appropriate team members.

- Nursing staff should be trained and deployed in clinical triage, minor illness management, chronic disease management and health promotion by telephone and be able competently to give and explain the results of investigations.

- Doctors should manage their consulting time flexibly in order to respond to those patients preferring to consult by telephone.

- Doctors should consider telephone follow-up as an alternative to some face-to-face consultations for common conditions such as depression and cancer.

- Practice teams and out-of-hours service providers should include aspects of telephone consultation in their clinical governance activities.

---

skills necessary for safe telephone consulting. When minor illness management is removed from the GP's workload, they tend to spend more time with patients who have multiple or complex problems, such as chronic disease.[83] It is difficult to determine from the literature whether the growing use of telephone consultation has caused greater demand from patients or has developed in response to that demand.

Changes in society such as the disintegration of the extended family, the wider availability of and easier access to health information, and the lower power differential between professionals and their clients all contribute to the need for flexible, responsive, patient-centred and multi-disciplinary primary care services. The almost universal ownership of mobile telephones reflects the contemporary need for availability and spontaneity with respect to communication. These social and technological changes have been reflected in NHS policy, in particular in the diversity of modalities of primary care provision now in operation in the NHS to improve access.[84] Box 1.1 contains guidance for practice teams based on the content of this chapter.

Exercises

Readers are now invited to take part in two exercises to determine their starting point with respect to telephone consultation and to develop Personal Development Plans (PDPs). Exercises appear at the end of each chapter accompanied by learning objectives so that readers can build a portfolio of skills in telephone communication and management – both clinical and organisational.

Exercise 1

Objective: to raise self-awareness of attitudes towards telephone consultation

The history of telephone use in primary care has shown that attitudes change with time and differ both within and between health professional groups, and between patients and their clinicians. Look at the sets of descriptors in Table 1.1 and decide which applies to you. You may recognise characteristics and attitudes in more than one set. If you feel brave, ask a trusted colleague into which category he or she feels you fit.

Table 1.1: Sets of descriptors

Set 1

- Comfortable with receiving and making telephone calls about a variety of problems
- Encourages patients to use different communication media
- Trusts own history-taking skills; rarely relies on physical examination
- Ensures patient's concerns are elicited and addressed
- Collaborative approach to decision-making
- Flexible in use of time during the working day
- Delegates work appropriately to clinical colleagues and makes use of administrative staff's skills and time
- Gives patients responsibility for the day-to-day management of their problems
- Shares limitations and benefits of telephone consultation with patients
- Tolerates the lack of visual and non-verbal cues when consulting by telephone

Set 2

- Receives telephone calls about urgent medical matters and makes calls when important information needs to be conveyed
- Prefers patients to make contact via receptionists or secretary
- Often uses physical examination to confirm history or reassure patient
- Relies on comprehensive functional enquiry when consulting by telephone
- Takes the lead in prescribing and referral decisions
- Groups telephone consultations in one block of time
- Maintains clear boundaries between the tasks appropriate for medical, nursing and administrative staff
- Takes personal responsibility for the day-to-day management of patients
- Unwilling to share uncertainty with patients
- Has a low threshold for bringing patients in to surgery when triaging by telephone

Table 1.1 (continued)

Set 3

- Believes patients get a second-class service on the telephone

- Concerned that the relationship with the patient cannot be developed over the telephone

- Relies on eye contact and physical touch in the consultation

- Acknowledges that the telephone does not support techniques like silence or nodding

- Flexible about consultation length

- Believes patients need time in the waiting room to prepare for their consultation

- Uses telephone primarily to 'buzz' reception or a colleague

- Prefers to work longer hours than to triage people away

- Reduces uncertainty by spending more time listening to patients

- Unsure about confidentiality issues with telephone consultations

Set 4

- Runs appointments at full capacity with face-to-face consultations and home visits

- Believes telephone consultations generate more demand

- Cannot convey authority by telephone

- Prefers to direct patients to leaflets or the pharmacist for advice about self-limiting illnesses

- Resistant to change

- Rigid starting and finishing times at work

- Dislikes being disturbed with telephone calls between surgeries

- Tends not to attend or contribute to meetings when patients' problems are discussed

- Rarely feels uncertain

- Regards A&E departments and out-of-hours services as appropriate back-up for patients

Exercise 2

Objective: to develop a PDP in telephone consultation and management.

Now that you have determined your starting point, the next task is to decide how you wish to develop in your use of the telephone in your work. Table 1.2 lists ideas for possible learning and development objectives and methods but you may identify additional or alternative needs. Record your plan and update it as you progress.

Any measurement you make, survey you conduct or change you make in your practice will have an impact on your patients and colleagues. Therefore it is essential to discuss your plans with the practice team. Receptionists are likely to be interested in what the patients think about their telephone-answering and appointment-making role so should be included in any enquiry about access. Senior clinicians with well-established habits may be less willing to experiment with new ways of using the telephone compared with GP registrars or a recently appointed practice nurse. Changes involving patients or their care should be thought through from

Table 1.2: Ideas for learning and development objectives and methods

Objective	Method
To understand the history of telephone use in my practice	Search on computerised patient database: review medical records over the past 10 years and calculate the ratio of telephone to face-to-face contacts each year
To assess the accessibility of the practice to telephone callers	Telephone survey of a sample of callers: determine how many times patients and carers try the practice telephone number and how long they have to wait for a reply
To find out what the patients think about telephone consultations	Postal questionnaire of a sample of patients: establish how popular among patients is the telephone for triage, advice, test results, follow-up and counselling
To understand the attitudes of the practice team to telephone consultations	Present a paper on telephone consultations at a clinical governance meeting or journal club. In the discussion weigh up the factors that would facilitate and inhibit change towards development of telephone use
To set up a telephone triage system in the practice	Involve all stakeholders in early discussions and start with a small pilot. Liaise with practice manager for issues such as staff hours, costs and impact on existing services. Sketch out a plan with the headings Who? When? Where? and What? or Strengths, Weaknesses, Opportunities and Threats
To audit the safety and effectiveness of the triage system	Identify patients who were appropriately managed by telephone and appropriately invited for a face-to-face consultation. Review critical incidents such as complaints or missed diagnoses in detail
To introduce telephone follow-up for patients with a named chronic condition	Identify a chronic disease from the Quality and Outcomes Framework for which follow-up data is required. Design a paperless call/recall system so that patients can be contacted by telephone and offered a choice of review methods
To reflect on and enhance my telephone communication skills	Ideally record telephone consultations with patients' consent and have a colleague or appraiser listen to some with you outside surgery time. Otherwise have a colleague sit with you while you consult, the telephone being used in hands-free or speakerphone mode. Choose one or two skills[85] to work on at a time from the following and have your colleague use a validated feedback method such as SET-GO:[85,86] • establishing identity of caller and whether he or she is able to talk openly • introducing yourself and your role • active listening • summarising • expressing empathy • eliciting concerns • explanation of symptoms and diagnoses, giving information in small chunks, checking understanding as you go • shared decision-making • safety-netting

their point of view, either by asking a panel of expert patients, or finding out how other practices have introduced a similar change. A useful tool to establish whether your practice has any problems with access is the General Practice Assessment Questionnaire developed by the National Primary Care Research and Development Centre in Manchester (www.gpaq.info/ [accessed November 2006]).[87] This is an approved method of gathering information for the Patient Experience section of the Quality and Outcomes Framework of the new GMS contract.

References

1. Anon. Practice by telephone. *The Lancet* 1879;**819**.
2. Toon PD. Using telephones in primary care (editorial). *British Medical Journal* 2002;**324**:1230–1.
3. Pencheon D. NHS Direct: managing demand. *British Medical Journal* 1998;**316**:215–16.
4. Loudon I, Horder J and Webster C, eds. *General Practice under the National Health Service, 1948–1997 – The first fifty years*. Oxford: Clarendon Press, 1998.
5. British Medical Journal. The telephone in general practice (editorial). *British Medical Journal* 1978;**2**:1106.
6. Hallam L. You've got a lot to answer for, Mr Bell. A review of the use of the telephone in primary care. *Family Practice* 1989;**6**:47–57.
7. Terry K. Nonbillables: when should patients pay for them? (editorial). *Medical Economics* 2003;**80**:58–67.
8. Office of Population Censuses and Surveys. *General Household Survey, 1985*. London: HMSO, 1987.
9. London Health Planning Consortium (Acheson Committee). *Primary Health Care in Inner London: Report of a study group*. London: DHSS, 1981.
10. Allsop J and May A. *Telephone Access to GPs: A study of London*. London: King's Fund, 1985.
11. Hallam L. Organisation of telephone services and patients' access to doctors by telephone in general practice. *British Medical Journal* 1991;**302**:629–32.
12. Hallam L. Access to general practice and general practitioners by telephone: the patient's view. *British Journal of General Practice* 1993;**43**:331–5.
13. Allen D, Leavey R and Marks B. Survey of patients' satisfaction with access to general practitioners. *Journal of the Royal College of General Practitioners* 1988;**38**:163–5.
14. Hallam L. Patient access to general practitioners by telephone: the doctor's view. *British Journal of General Practice* 1992;**42**:186–9.
15. de Groot R, de Haan J, Bosveld H, Nijland A and Meyboom-de Jong B. The implementation of a call-back system reduced the doctor's workload, and improves accessibility by telephone in general practice. *Family Practice* 2002;**19**:516–19.
16. Charles-Jones H, May C, Latimer J and Roland M. Telephone triage by nurses in primary care: what is it for and what are the consequences likely to be? *Journal of Health Services Research and Policy* 2003;**8**:154–9.
17. Brimberry R. Vaccination of high-risk patients for influenza: a comparison of telephone and mail reminder methods. *Journal of Family Practice* 1988;**26**:397–400.
18. Hull S, Hagdrup N, Hart B, Griffiths C and Hennessy E. Boosting uptake of influenza immunisation: a randomised controlled trial of telephone appointing in general practice. *British Journal of General Practice* 2002;**52**:716.
19. Quinley J and Shih A. Improving physician coverage of pneumococcal vaccine: a randomized trial of a telephone intervention. *Journal of Community Health* 2004;**29**:103–15.
20. Linkins R, Dini E, Watson G and Patriarca P. A randomized trial of the effectiveness of computer-generated telephone messages in increasing immunization visits among preschool children. *Archives of Pediatrics and Adolescent Medicine* 1994;**148**:908–14.
21. O'Brien G and Lazebnik R. Telephone call reminders and attendance in an adolescent clinic. *Pediatrics* 1998;**101**:1066.

22. MacDonald J, Brown N and Ellis P. Using telephone prompts to improve initial attendance at a community mental health center. *Psychiatric Services* 2000;**51**:812–14.
23. Piette J, Weinberger M, McPhee S, Mah C, Kraemer F and Crapo L. Do automated calls with nurse follow-up improve self-care and glycemic control among vulnerable patients with diabetes? *American Journal of Medicine* 2000;**108**:20–7.
24. Hagstrom B, Mattson B, Rost I and Gunnarsson R. What happened to the prescriptions? A single, short, standardized telephone call may increase compliance. *Family Practice* 2004;**21**:46–50.
25. Pinnock H, Bawden R, Proctor S, Wolfe S, Scullion J, Price D, *et al*. Accessibility, acceptability, and effectiveness in primary care of routine telephone review of asthma: pragmatic, randomised controlled trial. *British Medical Journal* 2003;**326**:477–9.
26. Hunkeler EM, Meresman JF, Hargreaves WA, Fireman B, Berman WH, Kirsch AJ, *et al*. Efficacy of nurse telehealth care and peer support in augmenting treatment of depression in primary care. *Archives of Family Medicine* 2000;**9**:700–8.
27. Meresman J, Hunkeler E, Hargreaves W, Kirsch A, Robinson P, Green A, *et al*. A case report: implementing a nurse telecare program for treating depression in primary care. *Psychiatric Quarterly* 2003;**74**:61–73.
28. Dietrich AJ, Oxman TE, Williams JW Jnr, Schulberg HC, Bruce ML, Lee PW, *et al*. Re-engineering systems for the treatment of depression in primary care: cluster randomised controlled trial. *British Medical Journal* 2004;**329**:602.
29. Marsh GN and Dawes ML. Establishing a minor illness nurse in a busy general practice. *British Medical Journal* 1995;**310**:778–80.
30. Gallagher M, Huddart T and Henderson B. Telephone triage of acute illness by a practice nurse in general practice: outcomes of care. *British Journal of General Practice* 1998;**48**:1141–5.
31. Kinnersley P, Anderson E, Parry K, Clement J, Archard L, Turton P, *et al*. Randomised controlled trial of nurse practitioner versus general practitioner care for patients requesting 'same day' consultations in primary care. *British Medical Journal* 2000;**320**:1043–8.
32. Shum C, Humphreys A, Wheeler D, Cochrane M-A, Skoda S and Clement S. Nurse management of patients with minor illnesses in general practice; multicentre, randomised controlled trial. *British Medical Journal* 2000;**320**:1038–43.
33. Venning P, Durie A, Roland M, Roberts C and Lease B. Randomised controlled trial comparing cost effectiveness of general practitioners and nurse practitioners in primary care. *British Medical Journal* 2000;**320**:1048–53.
34. Richards D, Meakins J, Tawfik J, Godfrey L, Dutton E, Richardson G, *et al*. Nurse telephone triage for same day appointments in general practice: multiple interrupted time series trial of effect on workload and costs. *British Medical Journal* 2002;**325**:1214–17.
35. Luthra M and Marshall M. How do general practitioners manage requests from patients for 'same day' appointments? A questionnaire survey. *British Journal of General Practice* 2001;**51**:39–41.
36. Nagle JP, McMahon K, Barbour M and Allen D. Evaluation of the use and usefulness of telephone consultations in one general practice. *British Journal of General Practice* 1992;**42**:190–3.
37. Wasson J, Gaudette C, Whaley F, Sauvigne A, Baribeau P and Welch HG. Telephone care as a substitute for routine clinic follow-up. *Journal of the American Medical Association* 1992;**267**:1788–93.
38. Delichatsios H, Callahan M and Charlson M. Outcomes of telephone medical care. *Journal of General Internal Medicine* 1998;**13**:579–85.
39. McKinstry B, Walker J, Campbell C, Heaney D and Wyke S. Telephone consultations to manage requests for same day appointments: a randomised controlled trial in two practices. *British Journal of General Practice* 2002;**52**:306–10.
40. Doublet-Stewart M. Telephone consultations (letter). *British Journal of General Practice* 2002;**52**:501.
41. Innes M. Telephone consultations (letter). *British Journal of General Practice* 2002;**52**:502.
42. Jiwa M, Mathers N and Campbell M. The effect of GP telephone triage on numbers seeking same-day appointments. *British Journal of General Practice* 2002;**52**:390–1.
43. Hallam L. Primary medical care outside normal working hours: review of published work. *British Medical Journal* 1994;**308**:249–53.

44. Buxton M, Klein R and Sayers J. Variations in GP night visiting rates, medical organisation, and consumer demand. *British Medical Journal* 1977;**1**:827–30.
45. Sheldon M and Harris S. Use of deputising services and night visit rates in general practice. *British Medical Journal* 1984;**289**:474–6.
46. Whitby M and Freeman G. GPs' differing responses to out-of-hours calls. *Practitioner* 1989;**223**:493–5.
47. Livingstone AE, Jewell JA and Robson J. Twenty four hour care in inner cities: two years' out of hours workload in East London general practice. *British Medical Journal* 1989;**299**:368–70.
48. Gadsby R. Telephone advice in managing out-of-hours calls. *Journal of the Royal College of General Practitioners* 1987;**37**:462.
49. Usherwood T, Kapasi M and Barber J. Wide variations in the night visiting rate. *Journal of the Royal College of General Practitioners* 1985;**35**:395.
50. Hallam L. Out-of-hours primary care. *British Medical Journal* 1997;**314**:157–8.
51. Cubitt T and Tobias G. Out of hours calls in general practice: does the doctor's attitude alter patient demand? *British Medical Journal* 1983;**287**:28–30.
52. Marsh GN, Horne RA and Channing DM. A study of telephone advice in managing out-of-hours calls. *Journal of the Royal College of General Practitioners* 1987;**37**:301–4.
53. Hobday PJ. Telephone management of out of hours calls. *Journal of the Royal College of General Practitioners* 1988;**38**:35.
54. McCarthy M and Bollam M. Telephone advice for out of hours calls in general practice. *British Journal of General Practice* 1990;**40**:19–21.
55. Department of Health. *National Health Service (General Medical Services) Amendment Regulations. Number 80*. London: HMSO, 1995.
56. Department of Health. *National Health Service (General Medical Services) Amendment Regulations. Number 702*. London: HMSO, 1996.
57. Jessop L, Beck I, Hollins L, Shipman C, Reynolds M and Dale J. Changing the pattern out of hours: a survey of general practice cooperatives. *British Medical Journal* 1997;**314**:199–200.
58. Salisbury C. Postal survey of patients' satisfaction with a general practice out of hours cooperative. *British Medical Journal* 1997;**314**:1594–8.
59. McKinley RK, Manku-Scott T, Hastings AM, French DP and Baker R. Reliability and validity of a new measure of patient satisfaction with out of hours primary medical care in the United Kingdom: development of a patient questionnaire. *British Medical Journal* 1997;**314**:193–8.
60. Leibowitz R, Day S and Dunt D. A systematic review of the effect of the different models of after-hours primary medical care services on clinical outcome, medical workload, and patient and GP satisfaction. *Family Practice* 2003;**20**:311–17.
61. Olesen F and Jolleys JV. Out of hours service: the Danish solution examined. *British Medical Journal* 1994;**309**:1624–6.
62. Hansen B and Munck A. Out-of-hours service in Denmark: the effect of a structural change. *British Journal of General Practice* 1998;**48**:1497–9.
63. Christensen MB and Olesen F. Out of hours service in Denmark: evaluation five years after reform. *British Medical Journal* 1998;**316**:1502–5.
64. Lattimer V, George S, Thomas E, Smith H, Moore M, Thompson F, *et al*. Nurse telephone triage in out of hours primary care: a pilot study. *British Medical Journal* 1997;**314**:198–9.
65. Lattimer V, George S, Thompson F, Thomas E, Mullee M, Turnbull J, *et al*. Safety and effectiveness of nurse telephone consultation in out of hours primary care: randomised controlled trial. *British Medical Journal* 1998;**317**:1054–9.
66. Poole SR, Schmitt BD, Carruth T, Peterson-Smith A and Slusarski M. After-hours telephone coverage: the application of an area-wide telephone triage and advice system for pediatric practices. *Pediatrics* 1993;**92**:670–9.
67. Department of Health. *The New NHS: Modern, Dependable*. London: The Stationery Office, 1997.
68. Munro J, Nicholl J, O'Cathain A and Knowles E. *Evaluation of NHS Direct First Wave Sites: First Interim Report to the Department of Health*. www.shef.ac.uk/content/1/c6/02/40/50/nhsd1.pdf. 1998 [accessed November 2006].
69. George S. NHS Direct audited (editorial). *British Medical Journal* 2002;**324**:558–9.
70. Sadler M. NHS Direct is value for money and improving (letter). *British Medical Journal* 2002;**325**:164.

71. Munro J, Nicholl J, O'Cathain A and Knowles E. Impact of NHS Direct on demand for immediate care: observational study. *British Medical Journal* 2000;**321**:150–3.

72. O'Cathain A, Munro JF, Nicholl JP and Knowles E. How helpful is NHS Direct? Postal survey of callers. *British Medical Journal* 2000;**320**:1035.

73. Marklund B and Bengtsson C. Medical advice by telephone at Swedish health centres: who calls and what are the problems. *Family Practice* 1989;**6**:42–6.

74. Hagan L, Morin D and Lepine R. Evaluation of telenursing outcomes: satisfaction, self-care practices, and cost savings. *Public Health Nursing* 2000;**17**:305–13.

75. Scarfone R, Luberti A and Mistry R. Outcomes of children referred to an emergency department by an after-hours call center. *Pediatric Emergency Care* 2004;**20**:367–72.

76. Turner V, Bentley P, Hodgson S, Collard P, Drimatis R, Rabune C, *et al*. Telephone triage in Western Australia. *The Medical Journal of Australia* 2002;**176**:100–3.

77. Wilkes L, Mohan S, White K and Smith H. Evaluation of an after hours telephone support service for rural palliative care patients and their families: a pilot study. *Australian Journal of Rural Health* 2004;**12**:95–8.

78. Ledek V, Deane F, Lambert G and McKeehan C. Description of a rural Australian free call telephone mental health information and support service. *Australasian Psychiatry* 2002;**10**:365–70.

79. Department of Health. *Raising Standards for Patients: New Partnerships in Out-of-Hours Care*. www.out-of-hours.info/downloads/oohreview.pdf [accessed November 2006]. 2000.

80. The NHS Confederation. *Investing in General Practice: The new General Medical Services Contract*. London: The NHS Confederation, 2003.

81. Department of Health. *Standards for Better Health*. www.dh.gov.uk/assetRoot/04/08/66/66/04086666.pdf [accessed November 2006]. 2004.

82. Department of Health. *National Quality Requirements in the Delivery of Out-of-Hours Services*. www.dh.gov.uk/assetRoot/04/09/12/15/04091215.pdf [accessed November 2006]. 2004.

83. Richards D, Meakins J, Godfrey L, Tawfik J and Dutton E. Survey of the impact of nurse telephone triage on general practitioner activity. *British Journal of General Practice* 2004;**54**:207–10.

84. Chapman J, Zechel A, Carter Y and Abbott S. Systematic review of recent innovations in service provision to improve access to primary care. *British Journal of General Practice* 2004;**54**:374–81.

85. Roland M, Mead N, Bower P and Campbell S. *General Practice Assessment Questionnaire*. www.gpaq.info/ [accessed November 2006]. 2004.

86. Silverman J, Kurtz S and Draper J. *Skills for Communicating with Patients*. Oxford: Radcliffe Medical Press, 2004.

87. Kurtz S, Silverman J and Draper J. *Teaching and Learning Communication Skills in Medicine*. Oxford: Radcliffe Medical Press, 2004.

CHAPTER 2

Communication theory in the telephone consultation

This chapter takes the reader through work on information and communication theory that has shaped current understanding of the consultation and which informs communication skills training. Consultation models that have been proposed or adapted for the telephone encounter will be described, and transcripts from real telephone consultations are used in the exercises at the end of the chapter to help the reader apply the theory presented.

Information theory in telephone communication

When speech is transmitted by telephone it leaves the speaker (source) as sound waves, is transformed into electrical signals by the handset, or transmitter, conveyed by a channel (wires – or microwaves in the case of mobile telephones) and then converted back into sound at the other end of the line, the receiver. Lastly, the intended recipient, or 'destination', hears the message. At each stage, information can be lost, especially when a noise source distorts the signal. The system used to encode the signal must be identical to that used to decode it. Shannon was a communications engineer at Bell Laboratories (USA) in the 1940s. He developed this model together with mathematical formulae as the basis for engineering solutions to reduce distortion and maximise the amount of information conveyed by telephone.[1]

Shannon's work has been applied to the study of human communication in a broader sense, the constituent parts of his model representing the generation and deciphering of language, and the physical noise representing various factors that interfere with accurate transmission and reception of information from person to person. For example, social communication has been defined as:

- a socially shared signal system, that is, a code
- an encoder who makes something public via that code
- a decoder who responds systematically to that code.[2]

This definition encompasses verbal, non-verbal, face-to-face and remote communication via any medium. A simple example would be Morse code, a system of long and short sounds, flashes or electrical impulses, depending on the medium used. Each letter of the alphabet is assigned a group of two to four long and/or short symbols (dashes and dots), which are used to build up words and phrases. It is a 'narrowband' or one-dimensional form of communication intended for brief, unambiguous messages, and fairly resilient to the effects of physical noise. Speech on the other hand is 'broadband' in that its capacity for information transfer is high and multiple codes are used simultaneously. Low-level codes such as words with single and universal meaning, or simple facts and figures, co-exist with high-level codes that convey anxiety, embarrassment, love, impatience and humour. Some of these high-level codes are non-verbal and rely on supplementary signals to be successfully transmitted and received. 'Noise' in its broadest sense can sabotage the communication channel at source (the effects of anxiety or alcohol), transmission (hoarseness, stammer), in the code (language, accent, jargon), at reception (hearing impairment, background sounds) or destination (distraction, health beliefs, relationship with source). Information loss due to a language, linguistic, social or cultural mismatch between speaker and listener is referred to as 'semantic noise'. Effective communication through speech relies on maximising the shared codes and minimising the unshared codes, in the same way mechanical or electrical communication methods achieve this through the use of identical systems for the encoding and decoding stages.

The social psychology of telephone communication

This section considers the theoretical basis for the differences between telephone and face-to-face communication by considering the effect of removing visual cues in interpersonal communication.

Studies on linguistic content

The circumstances through which communication takes place affects the ability of each party in a two-way conversation to identify and use shared codes. Experimental psychologists in France studied the content of the communication between pairs of volunteers under four conditions: face-to-face, back-to-back, side-by-side, and face-to-face but separated by a screen.[3] The linguistic content of the dialogue was analysed and it was found that pairs situated back-to-back and side-by-side used more formal, less familiar language resembling written text. The face-to-face pairs, whether or not separated by a screen, were linguistically indistinguishable, suggesting that psychosocial factors are more important than physical ones. Similar research in the USA involved pairs of subjects talking face-to-face but under a range of conditions: dark glasses, mask, mask with eye holes, and screen.[4] The method involved the linguistic analysis of the speech of both symmetrical (i.e. same conditions) and asymmetrical pairs. It was found that communication difficulties (pauses, interruptions) were associated with asymmetry rather than obscurity.

Studies on the outcome of negotiation

In a set of experiments that required subjects to take on the role of either a union or management representative, Morley and Stephenson (Nottingham, UK)[5,6] studied the outcome of simulated industrial relations negotiations under two conditions: face-to-face and sound-only link (separate room, microphone and headphone intercom). The roles were designed to give one side or the other the stronger case. In face-to-face negotiation the most common outcome was a compromise position, while in sound-only negotiation the most common outcome was that the side with the stronger case won. The lack of social cues in the sound-only experiment led to a more formal or impersonal style of communication. The full range of social cues available to the participants in the face-to-face experiment meant that interpersonal aspects could not be ignored. Inter-party concerns were therefore less prominent.

Psychological distance and cuelessness

Rutter (Kent, UK) found it difficult to interpret these results, because face-to-face communication was confounded with physical presence, which itself made available certain cues denied to audio subjects. In order to control for the effects of physical presence versus separation and face-to-face versus sound-only Rutter et al.[7] repeated Morley and Stephenson's experiment with the design shown in Figure 2.1. There was a difference in the degree of task-orientation, depersonalisation, spontaneity and outcome of negotiations between the sound-only groups (a) and (c) and the face-to-face groups (b) and (d), as if physical presence and visual contact had no significant effect. However, (a) and (d) represent extremes on a scale and when the content, style and outcome of (b) and (c) were analysed they seemed to lie in an intermediate position on this scale. The authors introduced the intermediate variable 'psychological distance' to explain the relationship between the lack of social cues and the subsequent content, style and outcome (Figure 2.2). Cuelessness is the term used by Rutter to describe the reduction in the number of channels used in verbal and non-verbal communication.

Figure 2.1: Physical presence versus separation and face-to-face versus sound-only

Separate room		Same room	
Sound-only link (a)	CCTV link (b)	Curtain (c)	Face-to-face (d)
No visual contact, no physical presence	Visual contact, no physical presence	No visual contact, physical presence	Visual contact, physical presence

Source: adapted from Rutter DR, Stephenson GM and Dewey ME. Visual communication and the content and style of conversation. *British Journal of Social Psychology* 1981;**20**:41–52.

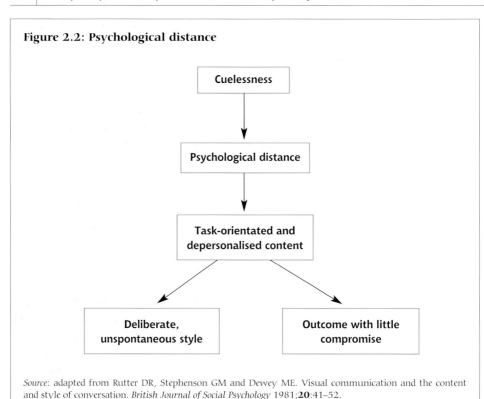

Figure 2.2: Psychological distance

Source: adapted from Rutter DR, Stephenson GM and Dewey ME. Visual communication and the content and style of conversation. *British Journal of Social Psychology* 1981;**20**:41–52.

Rutter's work also examined the effects of blindness in interpersonal communication.[7,8] Pairs of subjects (blind–blind, blind–sighted and sighted–sighted) were asked to engage in a socio-political discussion. Blind–blind pairs spent more time on personal information-gathering, less on the task, so their sound-only conversations were similar to their everyday experience, creating psychological closeness using skills that sighted people lack.

Social presence theory

Short and colleagues of University College, London (UK), described the phenomenon of 'social presence', a communicator's sense of awareness of the presence of an interaction partner and a variable in interpersonal communication that depends both on the medium used and the task at hand.[9] Media were ranked according to their potential for generating social presence:

- face to face
- video
- telephone
- monaural audio
- business letter.

Within any one medium individuals engaged in dialogue can negotiate, through conscious and subconscious verbal and non-verbal cues, the degree of social presence appropriate for the task, but within the restraints of that medium.

Clinicians' responses to cuelessness

Two experiments in a clinical setting illustrate how these concepts of cuelessness and social presence apply both to inter-professional and doctor–patient interaction. Consultations between nurse practitioners and remote hospital-based doctors using either television or conventional telephone were compared by Moore et al. (Harvard Medical School, USA).[10] In both arms of the study the nurse practitioner was presenting a patient who may have merited referral. Television opinions took twice as long as those given by telephone but generated half of the number of immediate referrals to hospital. The television may have allowed more social interaction and reduced the sense of isolation for the nurse practitioner. Conrath's study based on 32 primary care-based consultations in Canada involved doctors, nurses and patients operating in one of four communication modes: telephone, black-and-white television link, colour television link and face-to-face consultation.[11] Consultation length was dependent on case complexity rather than mode of communication and there was no loss of diagnostic accuracy with increasing cuelessness: all communication modes performed equally well. The style of interviewing differed, however, with doctors asking more questions of patients in telephone consultations compared with televised or face-to-face consultations. This led the researchers to conclude that doctors learn to compensate in consultations without the full range of communication channels by relying more heavily on those channels that are available. Most studies of telephone consultations have found errors in the diagnostic process, however, an issue that will be returned to in the next chapter.

Analysis of speech in the telephone consultation

Errors in verbal communication – either in expression or understanding – can have grave consequences in doctor–patient interaction, therefore both parties are taking a risk when 'language is always assumed to be in perfect working order'.[12] Linguistic mistakes can occur at one or more levels. In just one consultation transcript Skopek, a linguist based at Cornell Medical College (USA), identified communication problems between doctor and patient in the use of language (acoustic, phonological, syntactic and lexical) and through differences in knowledge, beliefs, intentions and interpretations of each party.[13] Spoken communication can be analysed on different levels. Linguistics focuses on the structure and function of language; it assumes that rules exist and that participants in natural conversation play according to these rules. Content analysis is a quantitative breakdown of speech into its component parts and eliminates some of the so-called 'para-language' aspects of natural conversation such as hesitations, pauses, overlaps and choice of specific words. Conversation analysis treats these aspects of speech as integral to the communication intentions of the participants, whether conscious or unconscious, rather than unimportant background noise. Conversation analysis 'seeks to describe the underlying social organisation – conceived as an institutionalised substratum of interactional rules, procedures, and conventions – through which orderly and intelligible social interaction is made possible'.[14]

The context in which telephone consultations takes place is likely to influence the pattern of talk because of significant institutional factors. Institutional interaction has its own 'fingerprint' of features[15] socially imposed upon the natural or fundamental domain of human interaction:

- participants have institutionally determined identities and goal orientations
- allowable contributions are constrained
- there are inferential frameworks and procedures.[16]

Communication theory in the consultation

One of the first comprehensive studies of doctor–patient communication was based on audiotapes of over 2500 face-to-face consultations conducted by over 100 British GPs.[17] In the quantitative content analysis of the tapes the authors described 37 categories of speech behaviour exhibited by the doctors that were grouped into clusters along a continuum from 'doctor's skill and knowledge' behaviours to 'patient's knowledge and experience' behaviours. The two extremes were later described as 'doctor-centred' and 'patient-centred' behaviours. Patient-centred communication skills in the medical interview are associated with more favourable outcomes, e.g. listening without interruption, screening and agenda-setting with greater accuracy and efficiency, attention to both disease and illness with patient satisfaction, and collaborative explanation and planning with adherence and improvements in physiological outcomes.[18]

Telephone consultation models

Patient-centred models have been advocated for telephone consultation by several authors; for example, Curtis[19] recommends the three-function approach:

- gathering data from the patient
- developing rapport with the patient
- patient education and motivation.[20]

Silverman *et al.*[18] were responsible for developing the Cambridge–Calgary Guide to the consultation,[21] the skills of which should be applied with greater depth, intention and intensity to the telephone consultation:

- initiation
- gathering information
- building the relationship
- structuring the interview
- explanation and planning
- closure.

Variations on the patient-centred theme have emerged through education and research. Table 2.1 lists the skills taught on a two-day course for GPs on conducting telephone consultations,[22] reproduced by kind permission of the course facilitators. The course has grown to include nurses and other health professionals, and is run three times a year by the Florence Nightingale School of Nursing and Midwifery and the Department of General Practice and Primary Care, Guy's, King's and Thomas's School of Medicine in London, UK (http://gppc.kcl.ac.uk [accessed November 2006]). The model includes many of the communication skills known to be associated with favourable outcomes both for doctor and patient.[23] The lack of visual cues in the telephone consultation makes it impossible to express empathy through non-verbal means (facial expression, touch) so it forces the doctor to make explicit empathic statements. Paradoxically the lack of visual input reduces the social inhibitions that normally control emotional expression so telephone consultations may contain more expressed emotion than those conducted face-to-face. This effect is compounded by the heightened anxiety associated with acute illness.

Table 2.1: Skills for conducting the telephone consultation

Stage	Skills
0 Preparation	• any available information about the caller? • anticipate time delay • note taking
1 Trust	• identify yourself • tone of voice • acknowledge caller's emotions • acknowledge caller's previous experience of health services • let the caller know that he or she is being heard • express empathy
2 Exploration	• question choosing open or closed forms • probe through reflection
3 Clarification	• caller's agenda • caller's understanding • reflect caller's statements back to him or her • summarise and paraphrase • allow time for the caller to talk, including silences
4 Action	• empower the caller to take action where possible • clarify what action you will take on his or her behalf • check that the agreed plan is understood
5 End	• when the caller feels heard, respected and understood • end the call for the caller not yourself
6 After the call	• time to reflect • note taking • other action

Source: adapted from Lambeth, Southwark and Lewisham Out-of-Hours Project. *Conducting Telephone Consultations. A two day experiential course for GPs*. London: Department of General Practice and Primary Care, King's College School of Medicine and Dentistry, 1998.

McCalister and McLean, GPs from Falkirk (UK), reported on the outcome of a Delphi consensus process involving 80 GPs and nine triage nurses in the context of their local GP cooperative.[24] The list of the components and actions of the telephone consultation agreed upon is given in Table 2.2, reproduced by kind permission of the

Table 2.2: Components and actions of the telephone consultation

Component	Actions
1 Pre-call assessing	• note apparent urgency • check if flagged patient • avoid preconceived ideas
2 Contacting	• give own name, whether doctor or nurse, and name of organisation • use patient's name and details • use appropriate language • be aware of tone, rate and volume of own voice
3 Information-gathering	• stay silent initially • ask open questions, then specific ones • ask about present problems • past medical history: filter questions, e.g. ever been in hospital? • ask the key questions for that presentation, e.g. if headache, is there a rash? • establish patient's usual health state and assess any recent change • drug history • social history • avoid third-person contact if possible • do not decide on management too early
4 Checking what the problem means to the caller	• ask about fears, worries, ideas and health beliefs
5 Clarifying	• check your understanding of problem matches caller's • ascertain the caller's agenda
6 Dealing with anger	• acknowledge it • check why angry • encourage caller to match own calm voice
7 Offering sympathy	• acknowledge effects of problem on caller and family
8 Negotiating management plan	• reinforce positive aspects of caller's self-care • agree to a visit early on during contact if inevitable to avoid potential conflict and use rest of time to assess priority • confirm understanding
9 Safety netting	• explain natural history of condition • give permission to call back if not settling or worsens
10 Documenting	• record accurately
11 Looking after yourself	• reflect on and discuss problem calls
12 Using resources effectively	• balance patient's needs and wants • be time efficient

Source: McCalister P and McLean K. A validated model for telephone consultations [rapid response]. http://bmj.bmjjournals.com/cgi/eletters/326/7396/966 [accessed November 2006]. 2003.

authors. Features of this model are the use of key questions, establishing how far the patient's condition has departed from its usual state (particularly important for patients with chronic disease and the frail elderly), and the early offer of a visit to prevent or diffuse conflict. These techniques will be explored in Chapter 7.

Car and Sheikh, researchers from Imperial College in London, conducted a literature review of telephone consultations that led them to propose the following approach, reproduced by kind permission of the *British Medical Journal*:

- answer the telephone promptly
- state your name
- obtain the caller's name and telephone number (in case the patient has to be called back by another member of the team or the call is disconnected)
- speak directly with the person who has a problem
- record the date and time of the call
- record the person's name, sex and age (obtain medical record, if available)
- take a detailed and structured history
- provide advice on treatment or disposition
- advise about follow-up and when to contact a doctor (for example, worsening symptoms despite treatment, symptoms failing to improve within a week, onset of new symptoms)
- summarise the main points covered
- request the caller to repeat the advice given (several times throughout the consultation)
- ask if the person has any outstanding questions or concerns
- let the caller disconnect first.[25]

If a decision is made to manage a problem without face-to-face contact, skills that have been shown by Curtis and Evens of North Carolina (USA) to reduce the probability of a patient consulting further are:[26]

- giving information about the expected course and duration of the illness
- describing signs that would indicate a worsening condition
- giving advice that is consistent with that of colleagues under similar circumstances
- allowing the patient the opportunity for further contact
- offering to address any outstanding questions or concerns.

Practical application

The multiple and complex process skills of the clinician are impaired by the limitations of the telephone as a communication medium. Through their emphasis on communication skills, the use of patient-centred consultation methods reduces uncertainty and shortens psychological distance. The absence of visual cues, the greater likelihood of expressing anxiety and anger, and the potential for miscommunication in telephone consultations conspire to make accurate clinical diagnosis

---

Box 2.1 Guidance on communication issues in the telephone consultation

- Ensure the mutual identification of clinician and caller, the latter being the patient whenever possible. This is the telephonic equivalent of a handshake and facilitates rapport-building, trust and social proximity.

- Gather information from the caller's initial message, the social context and the clinical history, with attention paid to cues from the non-verbal aspects of the narrative. Prejudging problems and early decision-making should be avoided.

- Address both the biomedical aspects of the problem as well as the patient's perspective: the disease–illness model.[27]

- Give a diagnosis or interpretation of the patient's problem with an explanation or a summary of the query the patient presents.

- Signpost the point at which a triage decision must be made (telephone advice, face-to-face consultation or referral) and involve the patient whenever possible.

- Negotiate the outcome according to agreed guidelines without pressure from workload or guilty feelings towards colleagues.

- Make follow-up arrangements for conditions that may require intervention or monitoring and providing a safety net to include worsening symptoms or other circumstances that justify further contact.

- Adopt strategies to enable the clinician to function at his or her best for the next call and to be professionally safe, particularly keeping good records.

---

and appropriate treatment decisions more difficult than in face-to-face encounters. Yet 'Effective telephone contact aims to achieve the same objectives as those that would usually be effective in a busy office, clinic, or emergency room. That is, to aid as many patients as possible in the shortest period of time, to minimise mistakes, and to be polite.'[28]

The 'Holy Grail' of telephone consultation is that list of questions with 100 per cent sensitivity and specificity, which enables the clinician correctly to distinguish between patients who require treatment from those who don't, reducing uncertainty to zero. Unfortunately such a list does not exist, but there are some key questions that might help in certain circumstances, for example those that establish whether the woman with pelvic pain is sexually active and the date of her last menstrual period, or the suicide risk in a young man who is depressed. The communication issues in telephone consultation and the models derived from research are summarised in Box 2.1.

Exercises

The exercises below include transcripts of real consultations. The language used by the participants has been reproduced verbatim together with its naturally occurring errors. Place names and the names of the doctors and callers have been changed in order to preserve their anonymity. Proprietary drug names have been changed to their generic equivalent. Table 2.3 explains the notation[29] used in the transcripts so the reader should be able to imagine the pace, tone and degree of closeness achieved by doctor and patient in each case. The aim of these exercises is to provide readers with an opportunity to troubleshoot consultations in the light of communication theory and telephone consultation models.

Table 2.3: Glossary of transcription symbols

Symbol	Example	Explanation
[	OK thank you [very much]	Onset of overlapping speech
]	[right then] bye	End of overlapping speech
[[	[[you go first [[you go oh alright	Simultaneous onset of speech
=	and I've got a high temperature= =Mm mm	No gap between speech turns
(0.0)	(5.0)	Length of silent gap in seconds
::	erm::	Prolonged sound
.	how can I help you.	Falling intonation
,	how can I help you,	Continuing intonation
?	how can I help you?	Rising intonation
word	she is *now in pain*	Emphasis or loudness
hhh	Yes hhh what er what strength are the nurofen	Speaker breathing out
.hhh	.hhh OK .hhh and does it hurt at the top of your jaw	Speaker breathing in
( )	Hi er my name's ( )	Transcriber unable to hear
(word)	Was there any cold or ear infection (or anything like that)	Transcriber uncertainty
(( ))	((laughs))	Description of non-speech sound

Source: adapted from Jefferson G. *Two Explorations in the Organization of Overlapping Talk in Conversation*. Tilburg: Department of Language and Literature, Tilburg University, 1983.

Exercise 3

Objectives: to reproduce the tone and pace of a telephone consultation using transcript notation and to apply frameworks from the literature to identify its strengths and weaknesses.

Compare and contrast the following telephone consultations about patients with sore throats. In particular identify the communication skills used and difficulties met by each speaker:

1. **hello?**
2. hello hi it's Doctor Cross here,
3. **hi erm yes um my erm fiancée she's um she's got this shooting like pain through her head and acute sore throat and and and glands all swollen I don't know what=**
4. =is she able to swallow.
5. **sorry?**
6. is she able to swallow?
7. **are you able to swallow. ((patient speaking in background)) she is but it hurts=**
8. =it hurts does it alright will you have a look into her throat there and tell me what you see right at the back,
9. **look in her throat?**
10. yeah get her to open her mouth really wide and look down the back and tell me what you see
11. **open wide (   ) erm its dark I can't really see anything**
12. alright ok look you you're in (   ) street you're not too far away can you come out to the Community Hospital there?
13. **where's that.**
14. er down Chestnut Lane your fiancée probably knows where it is er=
15. **=Chestnut Lane**
16. yeah you come across past High Road Surgery ok down High Road straight through the traffic lights and Chestnut Lane's the connecting road on the far side.
17. **yeah I know that.**
18. go down there about a hundred yards a hundred two hundred yards on your right hand side and you'll just see two yellow brick pillars and we're in there on the right hand side.
19. **ok then.**
20. alright then.
21. **thank you.**
22. anytime you want.
23. **ok.**
24. bye.

1. **Hello?**
2. hello is that Mister Scott.
3. **Yep,**
4. it's Doctor Dawkins here how can I help you.
5. **hi um I shh I I've been in bed since Friday evening=**
6. =mm mm?=
7. **=and sleeping constantly er=**
8. =mm mm?=
9. **=and I've got a high temperature=**
10. =mm mm?
11. **and the back of my throat is really really sore and it really hurts when I swallow or eat.**
12. right,
13. **and I've not eaten because it hurts so much and I just can't stop sweating and whenever I stand up I've got quite a bad headache but it's alright when I'm laid down.**
14. right so basically you've got a really bad sore throat and a temperature.
15. **mm mm,**
16. ok (0.5) otherwise fit well and healthy?
17. **yeah.**
18. take any regular medication?
19. **no I feel a bit when I stand up I feel a tiny bit dizzy and weak but=**
20. =right and have you been taking paracetamol ibuprofen,
21. **yeah I have I have**
22. and does that help at all?
23. **not particularly.**
24. we've got an emergency surgery at the Community Hospital if you've got someone if someone could bring you down we'll certainly have a look at you=
25. **=right=**
26. =obviously a lot of these things are viral infections and it's simple measures is all we can really advise but we're happy we'll happily see you.
27. **ok whereabouts is the hospital?**
28. it's on Chestnut Lane it runs between Main Road and High Street.
29. **right ok that's High Street (   ).**
30. yeah just follow the signs to the emergency surgery.
31. **and I just follow (   ).**
32. yeah.
33. **alright ok.**
34. alright then bye bye.
35. **bye.**

Exercise 4

Objectives: to reproduce the tone and pace of a telephone consultation using transcript notation and to apply social communication theory to its content.

Use the following transcripts to explore the concepts of psychological distance and social presence. Both callers are consulting about injuries.

1. **hello?**
2. hello it's Doctor Smith what's your problem.
3. **yes hello um it's about my four-year-old son.**
4. yep.
5. **erm he was swinging on um the swing and fell about three feet=**
6. =mm=
7. **=and landed on his stomach on um the edge of a trampoline erm and he's been hysterical.**
8. really=
9. **=complaining of pain he's been sick but he's just gone to sleep and I just wanted to know whether he may have damaged himself or just winded really?**
10. well he could have been has he wee'd since he did it?
11. **no.**
12. no.
13. **it was about an hour=**
14. =right=
15. **=over an hour,**
16. ok and did you give him calpol or he just fell asleep.
17. **I give him calpol but he was sick shortly afterwards,**
18. right ok and he probably just exhausted himself.
19. **yeah.**
20. right well we probably ought to have a look at him.
21. **ok,**
22. do you want to bring him up if you leave him asleep for a little bit then bring him up.
23. **ok.**
24. and if he wees could you collect it in a pot if possible.
25. **right yes that's fine.**
26. ok well I'll see you when you get here.
27. **ok thanks.**
28. bye.
29. **bye bye.**

1. **hello?**

2. hello is that Sandra?

3. **yeah,**

4. Doctor Jones here.

5. **hi.**

6. I got your story so you fell off your bicycle,

7. **yeah I went um over the handlebars.**

8. [[yeah I've done it myself]

9. **[[(   )] my kneecap.**

10. right,

11. **it um 'cause it flips out all the time it's quite normal.**

12. right so that's normal for you sort of dislocated [kneecap.]

13. **   [yeah and] I just manage to I just (kick) it and flip it back in.**

14. right

15. **but erm it won't bend it won't let me bend it (   ) I mean I've got it sort of with my foot underneath it at the moment ('cause) if I let it go really straight then it won't move a' all,**

16. sort of locked up.

17. **yeah well I've I can I've managed to loosen it but I can move it with my own arm it won't let my muscles move it's really it has actually swollen up?**

18. (1.5) ye::ah

19. **but I can't actually stand I mean when I sort of try to put my foot on it (   ) put my weight on it**

20. can someone get you down to casualty ['cause that sounds where you need to go so er]

21. **   [(   )] I live on my own I didn't know what to do so I thought oh I'll ring the doctor's but=**

22. =I'm not sure=

23. **=((sigh))=**

24. =that we can do anything Sandra in truth I mean it sounds like you nobbled it haven't you.

25. **yeah.**

26. erm its difficult to know for sure why you can't bend it but you've obviously dislocated it out and that you must have a lax ligament somewhere

27. **yeah [I have had   ]**

28.   [and the muscles] might go=

29. **=(actual) ligament.**

30. cruciate.

31. right. ((laughs))

32. erm.

33. but I mean I can actually bend it now by pulling my arm under it and pick it up it'll let my foot you know my leg will just bend now,

34. it might not necessarily be a good idea to bend it too much until we know what's going on whether you've torn a ligament or muscle or done something to the bone it's difficult to say but the truth of the matter is we're not really the right people I'm afraid ( ) erm I'm gonna have to leave that one to you how to I suppose there's taxi friends I don't know how you want to play it but=

35. =ok then.

36. hhh sorry about that Sandra.

37. that's alright.

38. alright?

39. thank you.

40. bye bye.

References

1. Shannon C. A mathematical theory of communication. http://cm.bell-labs.com/cm/ms/what/shannonday/shannon1948.pdf [accessed November 2006]. 1948.
2. Weiner M, Devoe S, Rubinow S and Geller J. Nonverbal behaviour and nonverbal communication. *Psychological Review* 1972;**79**:185–214.
3. Moscovici S and Plon M. Les situations-colloques: observations theoriques et experimentales. *Bulletin de psychologie* 1966;**247**:702–22.
4. Argyle M, Lalljee M and Cook M. The effects of visibility on interaction in a dyad. *Human Relations* 1968;**21**:3–17.
5. Morley IE and Stephenson GM. Interpersonal and inter-party exchange: a laboratory simulation of an industrial negotiation at the plant level. *British Journal of Psychology* 1969;**60**:543–5.
6. Morley IE and Stephenson GM. Formality in experimental negotiation: a validation study. *British Journal of Psychology* 1970;**61**:383–4.
7. Rutter DR, Stephenson GM and Dewey ME. Visual communication and the content and style of conversation. *British Journal of Social Psychology* 1981;**20**:41–52.
8. Rutter DR. *Looking and Seeing: The role of visual communication in social interaction*. Chichester: Wiley, 1984.
9. Short J, Williams E and Christie B. *The Social Psychology of Telecommunication*. Chichester: Wiley, 1976.
10. Moore G, Willemain T, Bonanno R, Clark W, Martin A and Mogielnicki R. Comparison of television and telephone for remote consultation. *New England Journal of Medicine* 1975;**292**:729–32.
11. Conrath D, Buckingham P, Dunn E and Swanson N. An experimental evaluation of alternative communication systems as used for medical diagnosis. *Behavioral Science* 1975;**20**:296–305.
12. Maclean J. Approaches to describing doctor–patient interviews. In: Coleman H, ed. *Working with Language. A multidisciplinary consideration of language use in work contexts*. Berlin: Mouton de Gruyter, 1989.
13. Skopek L. Doctor–patient conversation: a way of analysing the linguistic problem. *Semiotica* 1979;**28**:301–11.
14. Goodwin C and Heritage J. Conversation analysis. *Annual Review of Anthropology* 1990;**19**:283–307.

15. Heritage JC. Conversational analysis and institutional talk. In: Silverman D, ed. *Qualitative Research: Theory, method and practice*, pp. 161–82. London: Sage, 1997.
16. Atkinson JM. Understanding formality: notes on the categorisation and production of 'formal' interaction. *British Journal of Sociology* 1982;**33**:86–117.
17. Byrne PS and Long BEL. *Doctors Talking to Patients*. London: HMSO, 1976.
18. Silverman J, Kurtz S and Draper J. *Skills for Communicating with Patients*. Oxford: Radcliffe Medical Press, 2004.
19. Curtis P. The telephone interview. In: Reisman A and Stevens D, eds. *Telephone Medicine: A guide for the practicing physician*. Philadelphia: American College of Physicians, 2002.
20. Cohen-Cole S and Bird J. *The Medical Interview*. Philadelphia: Mosby, 2000.
21. Kurtz SM and Silverman JD. The Calgary–Cambridge Referenced Observation Guides: an aid to defining the curriculum and organising the teaching in communication training programmes. *Medical Education* 1996;**30**:83–9.
22. Lambeth, Southwark and Lewisham Out-of-Hours Project. *Conducting Telephone Consultations. A two day experiential course for GPs*. London: Department of General Practice and Primary Care, King's College School of Medicine and Dentistry, 1998.
23. Maguire P and Pitceathly C. Key communication skills and how to acquire them. *British Medical Journal* 2002;**325**:697–700.
24. McCalister P and McLean K. A validated model for telephone consultations [rapid response]. http://bmj.bmjjournals.com/cgi/eletters/326/7396/966. [accessed November 2006] 2003.
25. Car J and Sheikh A. Telephone consultations. *British Medical Journal* 2003;**326**:966–9.
26. Curtis P and Evens S. The telephone interview. In: Lipkin M, Putman S and Lazare A, eds. *The Medical Interview*. New York: Springer-Verlag, 1995.
27. McCracken EC, Stewart MA, Brown JB and McWhinney IR. Patient-centred care: the family practice model. *Canadian Family Physician* 1983;**29**:2313–16.
28. Brown JL. *Pediatric Telephone Medicine: Principles, triage, and advice*. Philadelphia: Lippincott, 1989.
29. Jefferson G. *Two Explorations in the Organization of Overlapping Talk in Conversation*. Tilburg: Department of Language and Literature, Tilburg University, 1983.

CHAPTER 3

Limitations of the telephone consultation

As well as the communication issues outlined in Chapter 2, consulting by telephone is beset with uncertainty on the part of the clinician because of diagnostic inaccuracy and a lack of training and confidence. This chapter reviews the literature on these deficiencies, initiatives designed to improve performance, and comments on the limitations of training. Most of the references are to American studies since the telephone has been used for a much higher proportion of consultations and hence has received more academic attention in the USA. The reader will then have another opportunity to troubleshoot transcripts of real out-of-hours calls from contemporary UK practice.

Deficiencies in information-gathering

Evidence of the quality of telephone consultations emerged in the paediatric and family medicine literature in the 1970s. Ott and colleagues from the University of Colorado (USA) assessed the telephone consultations skills of paediatric house officers with an experienced nurse practitioner playing the role of a mother.[1] In four separate recorded calls each, covering a febrile child, one with a cough, one who had ingested iron tablets and a call asking for advice about how to make a home childproof with respect to poisons, the trainee paediatricians were rated by two observers. The observers used score sheets derived from expert opinion and were found to be reliable. The authors found that insufficient information was gathered, particularly about medication already administered and drug allergies, and instructions about treatment were not communicated clearly.

In New Mexico (USA), Brown and Eberle[2] trained real mothers to consult about one of four fictitious but realistic sick children. The subjects were also paediatric house officers, some early in their postgraduate training, others more advanced. The completeness of the histories was proportional to the duration of the consultation but, again, key information was missing in most consultations. The mothers made qualitative assessments of the doctors and a common theme in their comments was the less than satisfactory rapport-building skills demonstrated. In the state of Washington (USA), ten accredited paediatricians underwent a similar assessment[3] for the same four symptoms of cough, diarrhoea, vomiting and rash, but there was no correlation in this study between call duration and quantity of information elicited. Crucial questions were asked less than half of the time. The more experienced paediatricians' telephone consultations were shorter than their less experienced colleagues and details relating to diarrhoea, such as state of hydration, or to cough, such as breathlessness, were frequently absent. The younger paediatricians fared no better in the diagnostic process but took longer over reassuring callers and giving instructions.

Health assistants in an emergency room (ER) in Boston (USA) used triage protocols covering 28 common paediatric presentations.[4,5] The content of the calls was analysed and compared with those of doctors and nurses not working to protocol. The medically qualified consulters omitted asking parents the age of their child in 18 per cent of cases, for tetanus immunisation status in 74 per cent of trauma cases and about the usual state of health of the child in 70 per cent of illness cases. The outcomes of their telephone consultations were also compared: 60 per cent of the calls in the intervention group resulted in ER attendance compared with 44 per cent in the control group. The protocols achieved safety at the expense of efficiency. The authors repeated the study in two primary care settings and reported that the subsequent face-to-face consultation rate was similar in the intervention and usual-care groups but presented no data.

Deficiencies in decision-making

Nurse practitioners performed better than paediatric house officers who in turn scored more highly than their consultants in a study from Rochester, New York (USA).[6,7] The cases presented to these child health professionals were a minor head injury in a nine-month old, a one-year old with a fever, a six-month old with diarrhoea, a toddler with croup and a five-week-old baby with projectile vomiting. A panel of 11 paediatricians contributed to a rating scale used to assess the instrumental or 'business' aspects of the consultations and the expressive or interpersonal aspects. The authors identified the phenomenon of premature decision-making in telephone consultations conducted by doctors, the 'mind snapping shut' at a point in the dialogue beyond which new information or parental concerns are ignored. Perrin and Goodman concluded their paper with advice on how to improve the telephone management of the acutely ill child: triage protocols and the use of taped calls from simulated mothers.

Two years' worth of out-of-hours calls were studied in a family practice residency training programme in North Carolina (USA).[8] Third-year residents handled most of the calls and 72 per cent were managed by telephone advice alone, with some variation between residents (60–93 per cent). As well as clinical and demographic data, the doctors were asked to record their emotional reaction to the calls. Twenty-eight per cent of telephone contacts invoked indifference, frustration or anger in the on-call physician. Such calls were associated with telephone-only contact and with problems of a psychosocial nature. A small sample of patients was contacted after the out-of-hours consultation for their views. A mismatch about the main reason for the call was found in one-third of patients surveyed.

Decision-making behaviour was studied among later cohorts of first- and third-year residents and accredited physicians by the North Carolina team.[9] In a quarter of recorded calls between the study subjects and simulated patients there was no identifiable diagnosis and in no call was there clear agreement between doctor and patient about the diagnosis. An inverse relationship between experience and comprehensiveness of clinical history-taking was observed, which led to a model being presented of the intuitive nature of decision-making for which a standardised educational approach may not prepare the doctor in training.

Yanovski *et al.* studied the decisions made by paediatricians and family practitioners at various stages of training in Philadelphia (USA) in response to simulated telephone consultations.[10] All of the faculty (fully accredited, institution-based physicians) were judged to have made the correct management decision for a dehydrated 11-month-old baby compared with about half of residents and private practitioners in both disciplines. The authors related this difference to bias within the decision-making processes of the different doctors. Community-based private paediatricians and family physicians operate in an environment with a low prevalence of serious disease. This may cause 'wellness bias', or an over-optimistic impression of the clinical case presented to them. Combined with the same 'shut-off' phenomenon observed by Perrin and Goodman, clinical errors are more likely to occur.

Training and confidence

Ten GPs from Cambridge (UK) were interviewed in 1997 about their experiences in consulting by telephone.[11] The doctors talked about their lack of preparation for this form of management when they started out in practice and expressed their continuing need for training in areas such as understanding the non-verbal but audible aspects of communication, evidence-based questioning and dealing with anger. GPs are more confident in their ability to conduct telephone consultations in their own practices during the day than when on call out-of-hours.[12] According to the 38 doctors in this study, factors most frequently associated with difficult calls are:

- difference of opinion on the need for a visit
- parental anxiety about children
- chronic conditions
- mental health problems.

Factors associated with satisfactory calls are:

- patient specifically wants advice
- patient agrees with the suggested plan
- problem is clear
- GP knows the patient.

Longhurst and colleagues sent questionnaires to 104 GP registrars in the former South East Thames region (UK) about out-of-hours work.[13] The response rate was 67 per cent and the main findings were a lower level of confidence in telephone advice-giving compared with face-to-face consultations in patients' homes. Moreover their perception was that the former management option is less effective. GP registrars who took part in the study found giving telephone advice anxiety-provoking because of difficulty in assessing the seriousness of problems from the history alone and in situations of demand on the part of the patient or carer for a home visit when this might not be necessary. The authors recommended role-play, tutorials, guideline development and greater initial supervision of registrars by trainers in the out-of-hours context as means to enhance confidence and skills in these learners.

Training in communication skills can improve physician satisfaction[14] and confidence[15,16] with telephone medicine. Confidence is also affected by willingness to prescribe over the telephone and availability of the medical record,[17] although the latter does not seem to alter the outcome of triage calls.[18]

Educational interventions

A training programme for paediatric residents in Philadelphia (USA) included the second of Perrin and Goodman's recommendations, taped calls from simulated mothers, and used small-group discussions as the teaching method.[19] The programme led to no significant consulting behaviour change over the subsequent six months. The authors raised the question of the purpose of the telephone consultation in acute paediatric practice: '[paediatricians] may see their immediate objective as merely to identify that patient who needs to be seen that evening and that a complete history, although valid, is not critical at that encounter'. Curtis described this process as 'parsimony in diagnostic logic'.[20]

Evens and Curtis (North Carolina, USA) reported on a comprehensive programme designed both for students and qualified professionals in primary care.[21] Simulated patients were trained to give a variety of histories, depending on the needs of the learners. The educational benefits of listening to and receiving feedback on one's recorded consultation were emphasised. Evaluation of the programme found it to be useful, relevant and valuable but outcome data were not published for another five years;[22] a cohort of family medicine residents that took part in the training were compared to a cohort graduating two years previously. The proportion of calls invoking a negative physician reaction and/or considered unnecessary was significantly lower in the 'trained' cohort. There was no difference in the proportion of calls leading to a face-to-face consultation.

Telephone TALK[23] was developed in California (USA) in a hospital paediatric setting but has relevance for British primary care since US ER staff of various disciplines see many of the common childhood health problems that usually present to GPs in the UK. This training and assessment instrument focuses on communication rather than clinical skills and consists of 22 descriptors of doctor communication behaviour. The acronym refers to the following:

- **T**rust-building – attention to the relationship between doctor and caller
- **A**ssertive interviewing – professional manner and interview structure
- **L**istens actively – picking up cues, checking understanding
- **K**ISS:

> **K**nows – confident but admits knowledge gaps
> **I**nquires – appropriate use of questions
> **S**olves – information-giving tailored to caller's understanding
> **S**trokes – supportive and complimentary.

Experts on teaching about communication in the consultation justify spending more time rather than less on patients consulting by telephone.[24] Specific skills include overt expressions of empathy based on what the doctor hears rather than sees through non-verbal cues in the face-to-face context, using the patient's or carer's eyes and other senses to supplement the verbal history, giving information in small chunks and taking additional steps to ensure it has been received and understood, including the repetition advocated by Car and Sheikh.[25] A framework for training is available that includes methods for developing appropriate doctor attitudes and skills using experiential learning methods.[26]

Consultation analyses

In order to illustrate the strengths and weaknesses of telephone consultation, three real transcripts are presented here together with comments on the relationship between doctor and caller, communication skills, decision-making behaviour and information-giving. Readers are referred to Table 2.3 (see p. 35) for an explanation of the transcription notation used. The first, about a 10-month-old baby, occurred on a warm summer's evening:

1. **hello the Hoopers.**

2. hello it's Doctor Jones here [you

3.   [hi=

4. =telephoned about Clarissa.

5. **yes thanks you um well I don't know=**

6. =yeah=

7. **=um and she's had a vaginal discharge and her breasts have been enlarged=**

8. =right=

9. **=for the last few days,**

10. yep.

Mutual introduction but no clear identification of caller as Clarissa's mother

Symptoms described in chronological order with minimal prompting

11. but just tonight I was bathing her and her left breast is um quite sort of lumpy?

12. right.

13. and hard.

14. yeah

15. and red and inflamed,

16. right [she's breast

17.   [and quite=

18. =fed is she?

19. she is yes quite different to the right.

20. right.

21. (   ) enlarged (   ) normal [(   )

22.   [is she distressed with it at all?

23. I wouldn't say she was distressed but part of the reason why I rung you tonight rather than waited until the morning is that I'm actually flying off in the morning with my sister-in-law to my sister's wedding.

24. right.

25. erm so it would be hard for me to get to see a doctor in the morning (0.5) um,

26. where whereabouts is your sister getting married?

27. Paris.

28. right (1.0) erm (0.5) hhh it's probably hormonal in truth.

29. yes.

30. um oestrogenic activity erm it can happen and as a result obviously you can get these other changes.

31. yeah.

32. um the pregnancy and birth were alright were they?

33. they were fine everything was normal.

34. and you're alright?

35. I'm fine mm.

36. and Clarissa's not got a temperature or=

37. =well I mean she's obviously hot but then we all are ((laughs))

38. yeah exactly,

39. um I wouldn't say she was terribly hot.

40. no.

Doctor's first question seems to interrupt caller's narrative

Effects of baby's illness on caller's plans given in response to doctor's second question about distress. Hesitation in line 25 a hint of her expectations

Doctor seems to have a diagnosis in mind but his attempted explanation is tentative and brief

Closed questions to elicit risk factors and screen for additional problems

41. **um it's just it's locally it's it's definitely infected it's so red and lumpy.**

42. oh I see you think she's got an infection.

43. **it looks to me as if it's infectious because it looks so different to the to the um to the right one it's definitely lumpy and definitely red um.**

44. right ok [erm,

45.   [er=

46. =well you can bring her down to the community hospital if you like I must say it's pretty unlikely in the extreme in truth=

47. **=ok.**

48. I I it's just where would it have come from of course erm.

49. **yeah.**

50. well yeah if you want to bring her down we'll have a look=

51. **=ok [ok.**

52.   [and we'll take it from there why don't we it's not going to harm her is it.

53. **no thank you.**

54. alright do you know where to come to.

55. **I do.**

56. cheers bye.

> Caller's idea about the cause of the baby's symptoms now emerges but met with scepticism

> Triage decision made reluctantly as caller's concern cannot be adequately addressed without a physical examination

Two factors, the caller's travel plans and her concern about infection, conspired to make the doctor agree to a face-to-face consultation out-of-hours. Referring to Perrin and Goodman's framework, there is evidence to suggest the doctor's mind 'snapped shut' in line 30 but it opened up again in line 42. The instrumental aspects of the consultation, such as information-gathering and triage decision-making, may not have been comprehensive but led to an appropriate outcome. The expressive aspects include good rapport, for example the light-heartedness of lines 37 and 38, but there are suggestions that the doctor needed persuasion to agree to a face-to-face consultation. The second consultation took place between a male GP and a 39-year-old woman on the same evening:

1. **hello?**

2. oh hello is it Jennifer Jennifer Potter.

3. **ah no it's her neighbour I rung on behalf of=**

4. =ok is it possible to speak to her?

5. **you can who's calling.**

> Doctor ensures he speaks directly to the patient

6. er my name's Doctor Timmins.

7. **ok then hold on a moment please,**

8. thank you.

9. **hello.**

10. oh hi yeah talk me through your symptoms it's Doctor Timmins hi.

11. **oh I've had nausea and diarrhoea since last night about eleven=**

12. =right=

13. =um I feel sick all the time at the moment doctor ( ) phoned up ( ) about six o'clock because I can't keep food down er I'm bringing up ( ) come out the other end=

14. =right=

15. =and she thinks ( ) getting dehydrated and she said try and keep doing the dioralyte and I'm trying but I can't I just can't do the liquid um um ( ) and she gave me some domperidone suppositories=

16. =yeah=

17. =to stop me feeling sick and nauseous I'm trying to keep them in but ( ) loo and my tummy ( )=

18. =right so just just=

19. **=( )=**

20. =so just to give me a bit of an idea as to the number of events have you actually vomited today or is it mainly nausea.

21. **no I've vomited about six times and I'm going to the loo about twice an hour.**

22. ok (4.0) and have you got gripy abdominal pain as well?

23. **yeah when I need to go yeah.**

24. yeah see any blood coming=

25. **=terrible headache=**

26. =any blood coming out of your bottom?

27. **um I haven't noticed any.**

28. right under the circumstances basically it sounds like a food poisoning I mean it may be appropriate to give you some ciprofloxacin antibiotics er did you eat anything unusual over the weekend?

29. **no I didn't and that's what I can't understand and I thought my children ate what I ate.**

30. yeah have you been travelling recently?

Open question to elicit patient's narrative and personal introduction

Patient refers to earlier consultation with another GP and subsequent treatment

Doctor starts a series of closed questions

The symptom of headache appears to be missed

Doctor offers his diagnosis and continues with more closed questions

31. **no.**

32. not been overseas or anything.

33. **no.**

34. erm I mean a number of different things=

35. **=the nausea I think that's the problem=**

36. =yeah=

Patient and doctor share their thinking

37. **=I can't drink.**

38. right it would be possible to give you an injection of an antivomiting drug and possibly consider giving you some antibiotics as well.

39. **yeah the only problem is I'm allergic to one of the ones for sickness.**

40. yeah.

41. **por chlor pror=**

42. =prochlorperazine.

43. **yeah.**

44. yeah what [about.

45.   [(   ) and it gave me a nasty reaction=

46. =[right=

47. **=(   ) violent spasms=**

48. =yeah=

Important information about previous adverse drug reaction

49. **=so I think that's why she gave me domperidone.**

50. yeah.

51. **(   )**

52. yeah that presents a bit of a problem doesn't it em you know what we don't want to do is to swap your nausea and vomiting for 'cause you see I mean any treatment for your vomiting won't actually help your diarrhoea.

53. **yeah.**

54. um and although you are vomiting obviously it is possible to get the fluid in in in amounts that will keep you going um I'll tell you the position we can offer to come and see you we can offer to examine you we can offer to give you antibiotics erm I'm not sure whether metoclopramide will cause you the same sort of reaction as prochlorperazine did.

Doctor runs through all the options for managing the symptoms

55. **right.**

56. we do carry metoclopramide here.

57. **right.**

58. um but obviously your erm what's called dystonic reaction you had with the with the prochlorperazine obviously that limits our choice a little bit.

> Doctor uses technical jargon

59. yeah.

60. so I mean er we could try some er metoclopramide as an injection and see how see how you get on.

61. can I do that? I've got to do something because I've got a funeral tomorrow.

> Triage decision made on basis of 'illness' as well as 'disease' factors

62. right I'll get a doctor round to see you er between now and twelve o'clock

The TALK team would give this consultation high marks for trust-building and assertive interviewing, and some for listening, but Dr Timmins missed the headache cue. In the KISS section his knowledge of drugs and problem-solving skills would be commended. The previous Sunday afternoon this female doctor was on duty and she handled a call from a postgraduate student with a Middle Eastern accent:

1. hello.

2. hello Doctor Dawkins here?

3. oh (hi doctor).

4. how can I help you.

5. erm I'm sorry my wife went out last night=

6. =mm mm?=

7. =here at college (0.5) and well she got very drunk.

8. mm mm.

9. er (I know) she has hangover but what worries me is that the veins of her feet they're very dark.

10. mm mm.

> Doctor uses non-speech sounds to indicate that she is listening to the story and the caller's worry

11. I can see almost all of them and they look quite dark.

12. yeah.

13. I don't know that=

14. =I think probably it's just that it's a very hot day you know and when it's very hot your veins tend to dilate and become more prominent than they are usually.

> Doctor's mind snaps shut at this point

15. oh [but,

16. [I can't think of anything else that would be significant really.

17. so it's I mean it's (not) important for me taking her to the (hospital).

> Caller provides a cue to reflect his concern

18. how is she in herself?

19. er herself she has terrible hangover.

20. yeah.

21. so she's not feeling very well.

22. is she drinking plenty of fluids 'cause you know you get very dehydrated when you drink too much alcohol and with the very hot weather she needs just to drink lots and lots and lots of fluid.

Doctor offers advice for rehydration

23. yes I'm giving her a lot of water and=

24. =yeah=

25. =( ) the thing is even if that it's hot er she feels cold in with her feet=

26. =right[( )

27.   [( ) dark veins (all) swollen some sort of circulation problem.

Caller verbalises his concern more specifically

28. mm:: I can't think it doesn't sort of ring any alarm bells in my head if you're worried and want her checked over we do have an emergency surgery at the community hospital.

29. ok.

30. and if you bring her down one of the doctors will certainly have a look at her but I can't think of anything too alarming that it could be.

Doctor attempts to reassure by indicating the lack of alarm the history is causing her

31. ok.

32. but you're very welcome to bring her down if you wish to.

33. ok thank you I'll wait actually to see of she over the (next) two hours (then we'll call).

34. right ok well we're here all day so ring back if you want her seen.

Doctor provides two safety nets: a face-to-face consultation or further telephone contact

35. ok thank you [very much]

36.   [right then] bye bye.

37. bye.

This transcript illustrates the effects of early closure in a telephone consultation: inadequate exploration of disease and illness, giving advice when the caller is not ready to receive it and unilateral management decisions. The lack of concern on the part of the doctor may reflect her own 'wellness bias'.[10]

Practical application

Awareness of the limitations of telephone consultation compared to the face-to-face clinical encounter should help the reader see the importance of learning new skills and emphasising existing techniques to maximise the effectiveness of inter-personal communication. The patient is equally limited by the lack of visual feed-back from the clinician on the line and may need extra help and support to convey a complex problem. Box 3.1 summarises the evidence presented in this chapter on common pitfalls in the telephone consultation.

Box 3.1 **Guidance on common errors in telephone consultation and techniques to help avoid them**

Errors in information gathering

Inadequate drug and allergy history.
Absence of key questions, e.g. state of hydration in diarrhoea.

Techniques
Open questions.
Triage protocols.
Checklists.

Errors in relationship-building

Clinician anger and frustration with psychosocial problems.
Patient anger over unmet expectations.

Techniques
Pick up and respond to verbal and non-verbal cues.
Overt expression of empathy.
Establish reason for call.
Supervision and feedback from call recordings.

Errors in decision-making

Premature decision-making.
Absent diagnosis.
Wellness bias.

Techniques
Frame problems in terms of disease and illness.
Include patient in decision-making process.

Errors in explanation and planning

Unclear communication of instructions and treatments.

Techniques
Give information in smaller chunks and check understanding by asking caller to repeat.

Exercises

Readers are invited once again to work through two exercises with the aim of developing analytical skills in the clinical management and communication skills of colleagues.

Exercise 5

Objective: to reflect on personal consulting and clinical decision-making behaviour through witnessing the practice of an anonymous colleague.

Read through the following transcript and comment on the quality and quantity of information obtained by the doctor and the appropriateness of the management decision. The patient is a 36-year-old woman and the GP is female. The consultation is taking place on a Sunday afternoon in June.

1. **hello?**

2. hello Doctor Dawkins here is that Missus Brierley.

3. **yeah.**

4. how can I help you.

5. **sorry to bother you erm (   ) I don't know (   ) I've got a chest infection.**

6. right.

7. **erm I feel it was two weeks ago I had an abscess? and I had (   ) it burst one night =**

8. =right=

9. **=it was bank holiday weekend I couldn't get to a dentist.**

10. yeah.

11. **it burst and I was very sick and bad and that.**

12. yeah.

13. **and then I went to I got antibiotics (   ) got antibiotics.**

14. mm mm,

15. **got it sorted out at the dentist temporarily till July.**

16. mm mm,

17. **erm then last Saturday I think I came down with this flu thing=**

18. =right=

19. **=um a week later.**

20. mm mm,

21. um and I've managed like dosing myself up 'cause I do twilights at the supermarket I'm not getting home till (   ) dose myself up shaking like a leaf all week in bed I've had all that I went to work today I said to the lady it's like on my chest and I'm not=

22. =right=

23. =(   )=

24. =yeah=

25. =a few packets of chips and I couldn't (breathe) go=

26. =right=

27. =down and it hurts all I want to know is will that be alright (or should I) ring in sick for tonight,

28. yeah=

29. =obviously I don't want to (   ) like this but am I alright to wait to go to the doctor's tomorrow or should I get (   ) now that's all I want to know really.

30. yeah are you coughing up anything?

31. yeah it's foul tasting.

32. yeah you probably ought to come down today and we can start you on some antibiotics.

33. yeah?

34. do you know where dutydoc is at the community hospital.

35. yeah 'cause I had to come (   ) bank holiday weekend about=

36. =ok

37. does it matter what time.

38. no.

39. (   ) car.

40. it's open till midnight.

41. oh right that's fine yeah.

42. alright so we'll see you at some time.

43. yeah alright then,

44. ok.

45. thank you very much.

46. bye bye.

47. bye.

Exercise 6

Objective: to reflect on personal communication skills that focus on the patient's illness experience through witnessing the practice of an anonymous colleague.

Read through the following transcript and identify the cues that reflect the caller's concerns and expectations. Which of these does the doctor pick up? The patient is a 63-year-old woman and the doctor a man.

1. **hello.**
2. hello is that Mister Smith.
3. **speaking.**
4. hi Doctor Cross here.
5. **yes.**
6. about Marjorie.
7. **sorry?**
8. about Marjorie.
9. **yes.**
10. erm I have a message here that she had a pain below her right breast going round to her back for one hour was getting sick=
11. **=she's getting a little bit worse she's now she can't move she can't lay anywhere she's crying her eyes out she's *now in pain*.**
12. when did it start,
13. **um I would say about two hours ago now.**
14. two hours ago and has she ever had this before?
15. **she has had the pain before and she visited her doctor and the doctor examined her and said he felt she was passing kidney stones (0.5) but I think it's a bit more than that now and it's er it's come on with a vengeance now and she believe you me she really is in pain.**
16. mm and is she very pale?
17. **she is pale but unfortunately we've just come back from the Caribbean to see our daughter get married and she looked she got quite=**
18. =( ) colour is she?
19. **she is ill.**
20. yeah.
21. **she's never ill this woman of mine and=**
22. =grand.
23. **and I'm worried.**
24. yeah.
25. **if you could get round here I would really appreciate it.**
26. alright then.
27. **thank you.**
28. ok.
29. **bye.**

References

1. Ott J, Bellaire J, Machotka P and Moon J. Patient management by telephone by child health associates and pediatric house officers. *Journal of Medical Education* 1974;**49**:596–600.
2. Brown S and Eberle B. Use of the telephone by pediatric house staff: a technique for pediatric care not taught. *Journal of Pediatrics* 1974;**84**:117–19.
3. Greitzer L, Stapleton F, Wright L and Wedgwood R. Telephone assessment of illness by practicing pediatricians. *Journal of Pediatrics* 1976;**88**:880–2.
4. Strasser P, Levy J, Lamb G and Rosekrans J. Controlled clinical trial of pediatric telephone protocols. *Pediatrics* 1979;**64**:553–7.
5. Levy J, Rosekrans J, Lamb G, Friedman M, Kaplan D and Strasser P. Development and field testing of protocols for the management of pediatric telephone calls: protocols for pediatric telephone calls. *Pediatrics* 1979;**64**:558–63.
6. Perrin E and Goodman H. Telephone management of acute pediatric illness. *New England Journal of Medicine* 1978;**298**:130–5.
7. Goodman H and Perrin E. Evening telephone call management by nurse practitioners and physicians. *Nursing Research* 1978;**27**:233–7.
8. Curtis P and Talbot A. The after-hours call in family practice. *Journal of Family Practice* 1979;**9**:901–9.
9. Sloane P, Egelhoff C, Curtis P, McGaghie W and Evens S. Physician decision making over the telephone. *Journal of Family Practice* 1985;**21**:279–84.
10. Yanovski S, Yanovski J, Malley J, Brown R and Balaban D. Telephone triage by primary care physicians. *Pediatrics* 1992;**89**:701–6.
11. Males T. Experience and perceived learning needs in out-of-hours telephone advice: interview study of ten GPs in a cooperative. *Education for General Practice* 1998;**9**:470–7.
12. Foster J, Jessop L and Dale J. Concerns and confidence of general practitioners in providing telephone consultations. *British Journal of General Practice* 1999;**49**:111–13.
13. Longhurst S, Shipman C and Dale J. Working out of hours: the experiences and training needs of general practitioner registrars. *British Journal of General Practice* 1998;**48**:1247–8.
14. Fosarelli P and Schmitt B. Telephone dissatisfaction in pediatric practice: Denver and Baltimore. *Pediatrics* 1987;**80**:28–31.
15. Males T. Improving confidence in out-of-hours telephone consultations: an afternoon workshop for GPs. *Education for General Practice* 1999;**10**:190–7.
16. Kenny C. Teaching consultations at a distance: three study days developed and evaluated. *Education for Primary Care* 2004;**15**:50–7.
17. Hannis MD, Hazard R, Rothschild M, Elnicki DM, Keyserling TC, DeVellis RF, *et al.* Physician attitudes regarding telephone medicine. *Journal of General Internal Medicine* 1996;**11**:678–83.
18. Darnell J, Hiner S, Neill P, Mamlin J, McDonald C, Hui S, *et al.* After-hours telephone access to physicians with access to computerized medical records: experience in an inner-city general medicine clinic. *Medical Care* 1985;**23**:20–6.
19. Curry T and Schwartz M. Telephone assessment of illness: what is being taught and learned? *Pediatrics* 1978;**62**:603–5.
20. Curtis P. The practice of medicine on the telephone (editorial). *Journal of General Internal Medicine* 1988;**3**:294–6.
21. Evens S and Curtis P. Using patient-simulators to teach telephone communication skills to health professionals. *Journal of Medical Education* 1983;**58**:894–8.
22. Fleming M, Skochelak S, Curtis P and Evens S. Evaluating the effectiveness of a telephone medicine curriculum. *Medical Care* 1988;**26**:211–16.
23. Kosower E, Inkelis SH and Seidel JS. Telephone T.A.L.K.: a telephone communication program. *Pediatric Emergency Care* 1991;**7**:76–9.
24. Silverman J, Kurtz S and Draper J. *Skills for Communicating with Patients.* Oxford: Radcliffe Medical Press, 2004.
25. Car J and Sheikh A. Telephone consultations. *British Medical Journal* 2003;**326**:966–9.
26. Stevens D. Teaching telephone medicine. In: Reisman A and Stevens D, eds. *Telephone Medicine: A guide for the practicing physician.* Philadelphia: American College of Physicians, 2002.

CHAPTER 4

Ethical considerations in telephone consultation

Transcripts of real telephone encounters have been used in Chapters 2 and 3 as examples of the consultation process. This chapter begins with the practicalities and ethics of voice recording. There follows an analysis of the ethical arguments for and against telephone consultation using the 'four principles plus scope' framework. This technique for analysing ethical problems was developed in the USA by Beauchamp and Childress[1] and has the advantage of being free from cultural, religious and political systems. The framework consists of four *prima facie* or 'standalone' moral commitments: respect for autonomy (self-rule), beneficence (doing good), non-maleficence (avoiding harm) and justice. The concept of scope allows the analyst to limit or extend the influence of one or more principles. The reader is referred to Gillon (Imperial College, London, UK) for a helpful summary of the theory of this framework in healthcare ethics.[2]

Voice recording

Devices are available that record the speech of both parties (or more in conference calls) engaged in telephone conversation, from tape recorders that can be fitted to an individual telephone receiver to digital recorders integrated with telephone networks storing many hours of speech onto compact discs. The latter types of recorder are commonly used by large commercial organisations that deal with their customers or the general public via the telephone. Many GP cooperatives use these systems but individual practices may find the costs prohibitive. Significant non-financial obstacles to recording telephone conversations are the ethical issues around consent and confidentiality, and the medico-legal risks involved in possessing 'best evidence'.

Ethical considerations

The General Medical Council (GMC)[3,4] sets out the standards expected of doctors in order to justify the trust of their patients. Doctors are required to respect patients' dignity and privacy, respect and protect confidential information, and avoid abusing their position. The GMC calls for greater openness with patients about matters of information stored about them and stresses the need for fully informed consent before disclosing information to third parties, even if the data is anonymised. GMC guidance on the making and using of visual and audio recordings[5] forbids doctors from making intentionally secret recordings.

Patients' interests, like those of clients and customers of other organisations that store their information, are protected by legislation. GP practices and cooperatives must register under the Data Protection Act 1998,[6] which became law in March 2000, and the Freedom of Information Act 2000,[7] which became law in January 2005. By these laws the patient must not be misled or deceived into giving data that will be recorded and stored. Patients have a right of access to data held about them, whenever that data was collected, superseding the Access to Health Records Act 1990.[8]

For telephone-based services the Telecommunications Act 1984[9] requires telephone system operators and users to be licensed. The licence instructs users to make every effort to inform parties that recording is taking place and to maintain a record of the means by which the parties have been informed. Written warnings in publicity material are acceptable means of informing callers and this is the position advocated by the National Association of General Practice Co-operatives.

Therefore patient consent is a key issue in the recording of telephone consultations. The current guidance of the GMC and the law make it clear that expressed informed consent should be obtained, but there are practical difficulties. In a study of telephone advice based in a London accident and emergency department prior to the changes in the law,[10] a method of obtaining consent was trialled briefly. Callers heard a pre-recorded message that invited verbal consent to their call being recorded and documented for the study. This method was found to hinder patient access, as the message took over 60 seconds to deliver. Hospital solicitors advised the authors that tape-recording calls did not require patient consent.

The argument to defend this position may have been that recordings of telephone calls to healthcare organisations are part of a patient's medical record, express consent for which is rarely required. This assumes that a recording of a telephone consultation serves the same purpose as a written record: an *aide-mémoire* for the clinician and a means to facilitate continuity of care and teamwork. There are two main reasons for recording telephone calls: to retain crucial information if contact with the caller is lost and to preserve a record of events should a complaint or negligence claim arise. These latter purposes are the more realistic since recordings are almost never listened to as part of the routine care and follow-up of a patient; rather, the contemporaneous written notes of the doctor on duty taking the call are sent to the patient's own GP the following day. Therefore the principle of implied consent that is applied to the written or computerised record should not be extended to the audio record of a patient's interaction with his or her clinician.

If practices or primary care out-of-hours services record telephone calls routinely, patients and carers should be made aware of this at the time of the call. Most general practices include information about their services and out-of-hours arrangements in their practice leaflets or on posters displayed in the waiting room, and, if applicable, this should mention voice recording. Even if such information is given, it may only be retained by a minority of patients and may not be recalled at the time of an out-of-hours call. Therefore primary healthcare providers with voice recording systems would be fulfilling both their ethical and legal duties by informing callers in the opening seconds of a telephone call that a device is recording their speech. A mechanism should be available to stop and delete a recording if the caller withholds consent to record.

Medico-legal considerations

Should a complaint against a doctor or nurse arise and medical records are examined, recordings 'trump' written records, which may be to the advantage of the clinician but not necessarily so. A parallel may be drawn with aviation disasters, investigators of which collect information from air traffic control records of communications with the pilot and radar data – indirect sources of evidence to explain the incident. The crashed aircraft may have a flight data recorder and/or cockpit voice recorder that contain first-hand evidence of what went wrong in the air. It is the quality of communication, contemporaneous written or computer records and subsequent clinical care that are most important in minimising the risks of complaint and litigation.[11] Recorded speech presented in defence of the doctor may not be admissible if the patient was unaware of the recording having been made.

Training considerations

Recordings of telephone consultations have been used for research and education as was explained in Chapter 3. The use of such data for these additional purposes also requires informed consent from the patient. Recordings of calls to receptionists and call handlers, and consultations with health professionals, can be sampled for quality control and training purposes. This requires the infrastructure and resources necessary to play back recordings, give feedback to or facilitate reflection by the learners concerned, allowing them to initiate changes that improve the quality of service provision (audit) or their communication skills. Transcripts of real telephone consultations or fictitious scripts can be used to develop roles for experiential exercises in a one-to-one or group format.[12]

Ethical analysis of telephone consultation

Irrespective of whether a telephone consultation is recorded, ethical issues arise when one considers that this form of healthcare delivery is prone to error compared with its gold-standard counterpart, the face-to-face consultation. What is the balance between the advantages and disadvantages to the patient? How can the rights of the patient be reconciled with the duties of the practitioner? The 'four principles plus scope' ethical framework helps in the analysis of ethical questions from four different viewpoints: beneficence (doing good), non-maleficence (avoiding harm), autonomy and justice. In healthcare situations there is often a balance between good and harm (e.g. introducing a new drug or surgical procedure) and between autonomy and justice (e.g. a patient demands an expensive treatment in a resource-limited system).

Beneficence versus non-maleficence

Those telephone contacts initiated by the patient or carer in which the caller expresses a need for telephone advice without wanting face-to-face contact should be 'good' for the patient concerned. Similarly those clinician-initiated calls to follow up a face-to-face consultation or *de novo* contacts for health promotion and disease prevention purposes should confer some benefit to the patient.

When a patient or carer expects face-to-face contact but subsequently finds himself or herself engaged in a telephone consultation with a health professional, the party who benefits rather depends on the patient's predicament and the degree with which the clinical problem is amenable to telephone management. A win–win situation is exemplified by the out-of-hours call from an anxious parent in a rural setting in freezing weather conditions about a febrile child. If an adequate history is taken and appropriate advice is given by the duty clinician and accepted by the parent then both are saved from a potentially hazardous journey.

Telephone triage is a demand management tool and, although it seeks to be supportive of patients and carers, the diversion of some callers to telephone advice without face-to-face contact is based on clinical experience and judgement, and is primarily for the benefit of the practice or out-of-hours provider. The organisation can operate more efficiently by adopting triage, channelling resources towards those patients with greater clinical need. Therefore the patient who is triaged 'in' to a service may perceive himself or herself to have benefited more than the patient who is triaged 'out'.

The avoidance of harm has long been a central tenet of medicine. Both patient and health professional are at greater risk of harm through telephone consultation compared with the face-to-face encounter. The patient is vulnerable to the adverse health outcomes associated with an inadequate or inaccurate history, 'wellness bias' and premature decision-making (see Chapter 3). The health professional who does not put himself or herself in the best possible position to make a diagnosis, and therefore provide appropriate treatment and advice, is vulnerable to complaint and litigation if the patient suffers as a result of his or her negligence.

Autonomy versus justice

Clinicians are required to respect the capacity individuals have to determine the way in which they conduct their lives. Patients exert their autonomy when they make a decision to consult about a symptom or problem and in getting involved in decisions about their care. Telephone medicine can both enhance and undermine patient autonomy. For callers with symptoms strongly suggestive of a minor, self-limiting illness or injury, telephone consultation helps to empower the patient or carer to manage the situation without hands-on involvement by a health professional. Both autonomy and self-efficacy are enhanced, and the experience of overcoming a health problem with some timely advice may affect the individual's future help-seeking behaviour. However, patients may be denied their ability to choose their preferred form of medical attention by virtue of decisions made by clinical judgement or decision support software in a telephone triage service.

Justice is a utilitarian concept that has enduring relevance in healthcare systems. Making the most of resources, both human and financial, is the shared responsibility of both practice teams and out-of-hours providers. The increase in resources in the NHS has not kept pace with demand and so initiatives that increase efficiency and cost-effectiveness to maximise the benefit to the greatest number are required for the sake of fairness. Because the principle of autonomy focuses on the individual and justice on the population, the two often conflict.

Some applications of the telephone can reduce health inequalities in a population while others can exacerbate them. Chapter 10 gives examples of telemedicine systems that help to monitor and support housebound patients who would otherwise not be able to access primary care services. Isolated rural communities use telephone consultations and telephone help lines to good effect, as described in Chapter 1, but the further a patient lives from an out-of-hours primary care centre the less likely he or she is to see a doctor.[13] The more resourceful, confident and assertive patients are those better able to negotiate telephone triage systems and may consume more healthcare resources at the expense of those who are less adept at expressing their needs. Social disadvantage is associated with difficulty in attending out-of-hours primary care centres.[14]

Scope

On balance, considering the convenience and virtual universality of telephone ownership together with contemporary multi-disciplinary, evidence-based and protocol-driven working practices in primary care, telephone access to health professionals probably confers more benefits on the patient population than risks. The potential harms can be reduced by training, good communication skills and shared decision-making. Justice may not be upheld if the quality of health care delivered by telephone is poor compared with face-to-face consultation. With the appropriate use of computerised algorithms in nurse triage and the integration of telephone and telemedicine services with traditional care pathways then quality can be at least maintained if not enhanced. Patient autonomy is important and it may be that telephone consultation has an overall neutral effect: it is an alternative form of healthcare delivery for the convenience of primary care teams (demand management) but an additional service for the convenience of the patient seeking information and advice (NHS Direct).

Practical application

A summary of the ethical and medico-legal issues with respect to recording are given in Box 4.1 and the main points of the ethical analysis of telephone consultation in general are given in Box 4.2.

Box 4.1 **Guidance on the ethical and medico-legal issues in recording telephone consultations**

Consent

- The status of or continuity of care in the multi-disciplinary healthcare team
    - it is stored for future reference in the event of a complaint
    - it may be used for audit, research or training purposes.
- Patients understand (i.e. give implied consent) that a record (written or typed notes) will be kept of their contacts with health professionals, whether face-to-face or by telephone.
- Patients do not give consent to have their conversations recorded verbatim by the act of making contact by telephone.
- Informed patient consent to record can only be obtained by a message at the beginning of a call, after hearing which the patient agrees to be recorded.

Confidentiality

- Recordings should be stored as securely as the written or electronic health record and should not be disclosed to third parties without patient consent.
- Circumstances under which confidentiality can be broken are:
    - disclosure in the public interest, e.g. in relation to crime
    - disclosure to protect the patient or others, e.g. children.

The GMC

General guidance:

- *Duties of a Doctor*
- *Confidentiality: Protecting and providing information.*

Specific guidance:

- *Making and Using Visual and Audio Recordings of Patients.*

The Law

- Data Protection Act 1998.
- Telecommunications Act 1984.
- Freedom of Information Act 2000.

Box 4.2 Ethical analysis of telephone consultation

Beneficence

Good for patients who:

- want advice only
- receive clinician-initiated calls.

Non-maleficence

Safety enhanced by:

- training
- protocols
- risk management.

Autonomy

Upheld by:

- greater choice (i.e. additional service)
- when health information is obtained
- when responsibility for self-care is handed over.

Denied by:

- less choice (i.e. alternative service)
- some triage techniques (e.g. decision-support software).

Justice

Upheld when:

- telephone medicine is integrated fairly into a healthcare system (e.g. out-of-hours providers, managed care organisations)
- limited resources are channelled to those patients who benefit the most.

Denied when:

- inequity of access results from social disadvantage or living in a remote area.

Exercises

The following exercises focus on operational aspects of a practice or out-of-hours service provider with respect to recording telephone calls and documenting their content and outcome in the conventional medical record (paper-based or computerised).

Exercise 7

Examine your practice's complaints procedure. What provision does it have for handling complaints that arise from telephone consultations? How good are the records made by the clinical members of the team when taking or making telephone calls about patients? Consider the advantages and disadvantages of installing a voice recorder in the practice to assist in the handling of complaints and for your medico-legal protection. Visit the following websites and enquire about costs and system requirements from the companies (all accessed November 2006):

- www.telephonerecordersdirect.com/
- www.crucible-technologies.co.uk/
- www.storacall.co.uk/svs_voistore_slim.htm.

Exercise 8

Design a system for obtaining patient consent to record consultations conducted by telephone:

- a form of words to be used by reception staff and call handlers to inform callers about voice recording of incoming and outgoing calls
- a form of words to be used by clinicians making outgoing calls to inform callers that the content will be both recorded as a patient contact in the written record and that the speech of both parties will be recorded and stored
- a method for recording in the medical record that verbal express consent has been obtained
- a method for ensuring that recordings made without consent are deleted
- a system of governance to monitor the adherence of the above by staff and the effect on patients.

References

1. Beauchamp TL and Childress JF. *Principles of Biomedical Ethics*. New York: Oxford University Press, 2001.
2. Gillon R. Medical ethics: four principles plus attention to scope. *British Medical Journal* 1994;**309**:184–8.
3. General Medical Council. *Duties of a Doctor*. www.gmc-uk.org/guidance/good_medical_practice/duties_of_a_doctor.asp [accessed November 2006]. London, General Medical Council, 2004.
4. General Medical Council. *Confidentiality: Protecting and providing information*. www.gmc-uk.org/guidance/current/library/confidentiality.asp [accessed November 2006]. London, General Medical Council, 2004.
5. General Medical Council. *Making and Using Visual and Audio Recordings of Patients*. www.gmc-uk.org/guidance/current/library/making_audiovisual.asp [accessed November 2006]. 2002.
6. Data Protection Act 1998. www.opsi.gov.uk/acts/acts1998/19980029.htm [accessed November 2006]. 1998.
7. Department for Constitutional Affairs. Freedom of Information Act. www.opsi.gov.uk/acts/acts2000/20000036.htm [accessed November 2006]. 2000.
8. Access to Health Records Act 1990. www.opsi.gov.uk/acts/acts1990/Ukpga_19900023_en_1.htm [accessed November 2006]. 1990.
9. Telecommunications Act 1984.
10. Crouch R, Dale J, Patel A, Williams S and Woodley H. *Ringing the Changes: Developing, piloting and evaluating a telephone advice system in accident & emergency and general practice settings*. London: Department of General Practice and Primary Care, King's College School of Medicine and Dentistry, 1996.
11. Medical Protection Society. *Keeping Medical Records: A complete guide for GPs*. www.medicalprotection.org/assets/pdf/booklets/records_gps_complete.pdf [accessed November 2006]. 2002.
12. East Anglia communications skills cascade facilitators. *The Telephone Consultation: A format for a pm teaching session for VTS registrars*. www.skillscascade.com/specifics/telephone_consultation.htm [accessed November 2006]. 2002.
13. O'Reilly D, Stevenson M, McCay C and Jamison J. General practice out-of-hours service, variations in use and equality in access to a doctor: a cross-sectional study. *British Journal of General Practice* 2001;**51**:625–9.
14. Shipman C, Payne F, Dale J and Jessop L. Patient-perceived benefits of and barriers to using out-of-hours primary care centres. *Family Practice* 2001;**18**:149–55.

PART 2

Telephone consultations and the primary care team

CHAPTER 5

The role of the receptionist/call handler in telephone consultations

This chapter focuses on the interaction between non-medical staff and patients or carers in both daytime and out-of-hours primary care. Fictitious dialogues will be used to illustrate the problems commonly encountered and to give the reader ideas on how to overcome them. The recommendations cannot be universally applied since the behaviours of the caller and responder will be informed by the unique context of the clinical problem and the operating procedures of the practice or out-of-hours provider.

Daytime telephone requests for appointments

The telephone network in a practice and its connections to the outside world represent one of several systems that help the organisation to function. The telephone system is configured according to the size, style and degree of development of the practice. A small practice with a low consultation rate and a traditional block-release appointment system may have one incoming line and a steady influx of calls that can be managed by one receptionist at a time handling appointment and visit requests, and other enquiries alongside non-telephone tasks. Outgoing calls may occur sporadically during the day with perhaps a small block of telephone consultations at the end of the morning surgery when the doctors view the 'message book'. A large practice in an area of high demand running a book-on-the-day system may need to open several incoming lines in the early part of the morning with as many receptionists taking calls from patients competing not only for the telephone lines[1] but also for the day's allocation of free appointments.[2] Nurses and/or doctors may simultaneously be making outgoing triage calls, managing some problems with telephone advice, some by cross-referral to a colleague and others by inviting the patients in for a face-to face consultation.

Reception staff members are the 'front end' of the practice and have a complex role that is rarely appreciated by the wider primary healthcare team.[3] Making appointments for patients requires social and negotiating skills.[4] Because receptionists act according to practice policies and within an appointment system they are perceived by many patients as a barrier between them and the clinician they wish to consult.[5] The confidence that a caller has in breaking through this barrier will depend on:

- his or her state of mind (which might be affected by illness or number of attempts made to contact the surgery)
- urgency of the problem
- previous experience of calling the practice
- understanding of the healthcare system
- level of education
- culture
- language
- ability to communicate (which may be impaired by a crying baby or being within earshot of colleagues at work).

A survey of receptionists in 50 practices in Leeds with a response rate of 70 per cent revealed that verbal abuse, both face-to-face and over the telephone, is a common experience.[6] Some patients get to know receptionists by their voice over the telephone and receptionists become familiar with frequent callers. It is important, on the one hand, for receptionists to be fair in their allocation of appointments to patients but, on the other hand, to help build and maintain the relationship between the practice and the patient population. Incoming calls should be answered with a standard introduction followed by a listening phase in which the reception seeks to identify what the caller wants. If the request from the caller is to make an appointment the response will depend on the appointment system of the practice.

Urgent or routine?

Some appointment systems only distinguish between 'urgent' and 'routine' slots where appointments available the same day are for urgent problems only. This combined system has proven to be acceptable to patients,[7] but the patient has to claim urgency if he or she wants to be seen the same day. If it can be established that the problem is routine then an appointment in the future can be offered. This requires the receptionist to help the patient distinguish between urgent and routine without the benefit of medical training:

good morning High Street Surgery how may I help you.

good morning I'd like to see Doctor Brown please,

the next appointment for Doctor Brown is Friday morning at ten o'clock is that ok?

oh I was hoping to see him today you see=

=I only have urgent appointments today and they are with Doctor Green

well I don't know if it's urgent

can it wait until Friday? two more days?

well I really need advice today because by Friday=

=so it's urgent then.

well=

=Doctor Green at eleven thirty and the name is?

Farmer Eric Farmer.

It is not clear whether the patient has been allocated an appropriate appointment because of the uncertainty surrounding the urgency of the problem. Some practices issue guidance to receptionists about what constitutes an urgent problem but more often than not it is left to the receptionist to use common sense:

good morning High Street Surgery how may I help you.

good morning I'd like to see Doctor Brown please,

the next appointment for Doctor Brown is Friday morning at ten o'clock is that ok?

oh I was hoping to see him today you see I go into hospital on Friday

mm mm

and they want me to take this form in with me signed by Doctor Brown

I see (0.5) anything else?

no no just the form

well why not bring it in and I'll ask Doctor Brown to look at it for you what's the name?

The reason for the call became clear because the receptionist took time to listen without interrupting and relieved Doctor Green of additional paperwork.

Book-on-the-day

The setting for the next example is a practice that has introduced Advanced Access[8] with a small proportion of appointments available for booking ahead. This system is based on demand management models from the US commercial world: efficiency can be improved, delays reduced and customer satisfaction enhanced by re-engineering the systems that govern manufacturing and delivery processes.[9] Its chief principle is 'do today's work today' through a process of predicting demand and matching capacity to that demand on a responsive day-to-day basis. It has been criticised for its impact on continuity of care and lack of evaluation.[10]

good morning High Street Surgery how may I help you

hello there I'd like to see the GP next Monday please

we have a book on the day system if you want an appointment next Monday you have to ring back then between eight thirty and nine=

=but it's so difficult to get through at that time couldn't I book something now,

I can make you an appointment for today what time would you like.

oh I shan't bother goodbye.

The unsatisfactory ending to this call reflects the conflict between the need or desire of the practice to comply with access targets[11] and the needs of the patient for flexibility. Practices are required to provide appointments with any health professional in the primary care team within 24 hours and with a GP within 48 hours.[11] Patients may override this requirement by requesting advance appointments that fit more conveniently with their lifestyle or physiology. Hanging on for more information can enlighten the situation and lead to a more satisfactory result for all concerned:

good morning High Street Surgery how may I help you.

hello there I'd like to see the GP next Monday please,

next Monday.

well it has to be then because that's when I come on.

I see=

=and Doctor White said the nurse has to be there too to help

did the doctor talk about the appointment system we are using these days?

not really but he said when I book in to say coils should be on the exception list

ok that means your situation is one where we book ahead but most appointments are book on the day

ok

what was the name please.

Practical procedures such as coil-fittings and elective minor operations are examples of appointments that usually need an appointment to be booked in advance. Practices may include categories of patients such as those who commute or work at night in a list of criteria for bypassing the book-on-the-day system.

Triage system

A variation on the book-on-the-day model is the practice that operates both Advanced Access and telephone triage. The receptionist's task is to perform a preliminary triage in order to book the patient straight into an appointment slot or arrange for a nurse to telephone the caller back:

good morning High Street Surgery how may I help you.

it's my wife I'm a bit worried about her.

what do you mean worried.

well she was alright yesterday then she's been sick and bad all night,

oh dear well I'll ask the nurse to call you back

but she needs the doctor=

=the nurse will decide that what's her name?

Margaret Matthews

ok Mister Matthews hang on a few minutes for the nurse goodbye.

Receptionists involved in the triage process usually benefit from using stock phrases that explain the system in a supportive way:

good morning High Street Surgery how may I help you.

it's my wife I'm a bit worried about her.

can you give me some idea of the problem so I can give you the most appropriate appointment.

well it started in the night she's been sick and bad,

I see do you mean vomiting?

yes and the other way too.

what do you=

=diarrhoea.

ok so it's vomiting and diarrhoea that came on in the night.

yes can the doctor come?

that's quite possible but what I'll do first is ask the nurse to call you back to take down some more details and then I'm sure she'll discuss it with the doctor.

when will that be I can't stay by the phone,

in a few minutes.

alright then.

what's your wife's name?

The receptionist should then alert the triage nurse about the request and might add a comment such as 'expecting a home visit' to give an indication of the degree of urgency or concern expressed during the initial telephone contact.

It is important that practices provide appropriate training for receptionists who perform a triage function. The British Medical Association's (BMA) General Practitioners Committee responded to queries received by the BMA's Public Affairs Division about receptionist triage:[12] some patients objected to revealing their symptoms to administrative staff, preferring only to express a preference for the clinician they felt would meet their clinical needs. These rights need to be reconciled with the capacity and configuration of the practice. Reception staff should know what sort of problems are dealt with by which healthcare professional and should have the communication skills to explain their role on guiding the patient to the most appropriate appointment.

The role of the out-of-hours call handler

Out-of-hours services (apart from walk-in centres, nurse-led primary care services in urban settings offering daytime and evening assessments, and accident and emergency departments) require patients and carers to make initial telephone contact with a message-taker or call handler. Traditionally undertaken by the GP's spouse, this role requires skills similar to those of the practice receptionist – indeed some receptionists supplement their income by handling out-of-hours calls for GPs on duty. Call handlers are required to take and relay requests for medical help competently. A survey of 91 primary care practices in Denver (USA), which used answering services for out-of-hours calls and performed a triage function,[13] found that a mean of 50 per cent (range 22–77 per cent) of calls not passed on to the doctor on duty were worthy of immediate clinical assessment. The survey concluded that the call-handling services under scrutiny imposed barriers that may delay care. In UK GP cooperatives and Primary Care Organisation (PCO)-commissioned out-of-hours services call handlers perform a brief triage function in order to help maintain NHS standards. This is in order to distinguish the emergency situation that would be better managed by 'blue light' ambulance service response from those that should be passed on to duty doctors and nurses:

good evening doctors' emergency service are you calling about yourself or someone else.

It's about my mother actually,

ok is she conscious and breathing?

well yes=

=which doctor is she registered with.

Signposting the triage function

Call handlers need to be aware of how these opening statements come across to callers and may wish to signpost the triage function or at least explain the reason behind the questions:

good evening doctors' emergency service are you calling about yourself or someone else.

it's about my mother actually,

ok just a couple of quick questions first is she conscious and breathing?

oh yes.

and are you with her?

I am.

thanks it's just that sometimes people need 999 not us.

I understand=

=which doctor is she registered with.

Taking the message

The message needs to include the patient's details, the caller's name and relationship if not the patient, the telephone number for the return call and a summary of the clinical problem. Unless the call handler is using an electronic database that automatically records the date and time of the call this information also needs to be taken down. Summarising is just as effective in the call handler's repertoire of communication skills as it is in the clinician's:

so that's bleeding from her bottom on and off for three days getting heavier tonight she's feeling faint and looks pale.

yes that's right.

and the address is Forty-Two High Street next to the Coach and Horses?

no opposite.

sorry opposite right I'll get the duty doctor to call you back on oh one two two three six six nine seven seven four.

thank you.

ok goodbye.

Relaying the message

The call handler then passes this information on to the duty doctor if working for a GP rota or deputising service or to the clinical team in larger organisations. The possible media for this stage are telephone, either direct or via a pager, written (printed if in a computerised environment) or through short-wave radio contact. Radio communication has its own unique convention, and information passed this way is not secure, therefore patients' confidentiality is at risk. A combination of radio message and fax or wireless remote printing facility is safer in services that have mobile teams such as paramedics or doctor/driver combinations:

dutydoc base calling car three,

car three come in dutydoc base over?

I have a visit for you may I fax it to you over,

go ahead over,

it's quite urgent could you start making your way to the High Street over,

roger dutydoc base proceeding to the High Street over.

thank you car three dutydoc base out.

Multi-tasking

As with all staff in the NHS call handlers need to be able to work well under pressure. Only one call can be dealt with effectively at a time and it is better to conduct each consultation thoroughly before taking the next in the interests of patient safety:

good evening doctors' emergency service are you calling about yourself or someone else.

myself

ok can you tell me which doctor you are registered with

Doctor Green at the High Street Surg=

=can I ask you to hold just a moment

ok

good evening doctors' emergency service are you calling about yourself or someone else.

it's my baby I need the doctor straight away

is your baby conscious and breathing

screaming his little head off

ok I'll take some details in a moment please hold on while I finish another call quickly

please hurry =

= I will ((returns to first call)) sorry about that what's the number you're calling from please.

Administrative calls

Lastly call handlers receive calls from patients who just need information about their own practice or reminding that routine problems and appointment requests are dealt with during the normal working day:

good evening doctors' emergency service are you calling about yourself or someone else.

is that the doctors'?

it's the emergency service for the doctors.

I need to see Doctor Green.

Doctor Green isn't on duty tonight.

but he told me to make an appointment for a blood pressure check.

the surgeries are closed now we're the emergency service?

well what shall I do?

telephone the surgery tomorrow morning the phone line opens at eight thirty.

eight thirty I see,

is that alright.

yes sorry to bother you.

that's alright goodnight.

goodnight.

Personal development for receptionists and call handlers

There are opportunities for receptionists to develop their skills either within the practice or out-of-hours service if in-house training is available or through clinical governance events organised by their PCO. Call handlers recruited by NHS organisations receive training in the early stages of their employment.[14,15] Nationally recognised qualifications such as those run and assessed by the Association of Medical Secretaries, Practice Managers and Receptionists (AMSPAR) require reception staff to be released for courses. AMSPAR offers a certificate in General Practice Reception[16] that covers:

1. Ethics, Confidentiality and the Role of the Receptionist in General Practice
2. Communication Skills, Patient Care and Discrimination Awareness in General Practice

3. First Aid, Health and Safety, and Legal Aspects in General Practice
4. Preventive Medicine, Control of Drugs, Repeat Prescriptions and Medical Audit in General Practice
5. Medical Terminology in General Practice
6. Stress Management, Motivation and Delegation in General Practice.

AMSPAR recommends several textbooks for reception staff among which is Robbins's *Handbook*.[17]

Practical application

Receptionists and call handlers perform a vital function at the interface between the general public and the primary care team they represent. Non-medical support staff should be supported in their stressful role of converting demand for appointments, information and relief of anxiety into lists of tasks for their medical, nursing and paramedical colleagues to work through. Box 5.1 provides guidance for receptionists and call handlers in their telephone communication with patients and carers.

Box 5.1 Guidance for receptionists and call handlers in telephone communication

- Be thoroughly familiar with the practice's appointment system and its rationale.
- Understand both the rigid and flexible components of the system.
- Appreciate how the practice meets the NHS access targets.
- Be thoroughly familiar with the practice's or out-of-hours service's triage system.
- Answer each incoming call in a standardised way, stating the name of the surgery or out-of-hours service, a personal introduction and an open question.
- Frame responses in the positive in order to avoid conflict and diffuse any aggression.
- Establish the purpose of the call as early as possible in order efficiently to complete the call or pass the caller to an appropriate team member.
- If the purpose of the call is not clear, consider reasons why the caller might have difficulties, e.g. lack of sleep, pain, language or learning difficulties.
- Express empathy to callers who are confused or in distress and be prepared to take extra time.
- In cases of doubt over the urgency of a problem, err on the side of caution but communicate your doubt to the responsible clinician and ask for feedback.

Exercises

Readers from all backgrounds are welcome to attempt the following exercises, which are intended to develop organisational skills. Although the scenarios below will usually be managed by administrative staff, health professionals also need to be prepared to solve logistical communication problems.

Exercise 9

Objectives: to assess an unexpected organisational problem and contribute to a team effort to rectify it.

You are the first to arrive at the practice one Monday morning to find that the telephone system is not working. The computer system is functioning and details of patients pre-booked to attend are available. In 30 minutes patients will attempt to contact the surgery for same-day appointments. There are two mobile phones available that are used by on-call doctors when they are out on visits. You use one to contact the telephone company to report the fault. The response is likely to take four to six hours. How could you help the practice manage the situation with minimum inconvenience to patients?

Exercise 10

Objectives: to develop organisational skills and facilitate effective teamwork under conditions of unexpectedly high demand.

You are working on a Monday evening for an out-of-hours service. The workload is particularly heavy from the start of the shift because a local surgery was unable to take telephone calls for most of the day. The unexpected number of patients comprises both 'walk-ins' and telephone calls. Most of the problems are minor but some require home visits. The service is close to becoming overwhelmed and unable to respond to urgent cases. You are aware of the targets that must be met for responding to patients. How can you help the service function under these circumstances?

References

1. Hallam L. Access to general practice and general practitioners by telephone: the patient's view. *British Journal of General Practice* 1993;**43**:331–5.
2. Windridge K, Tarrant C, Freeman G, Baker R, Boulton M and Low J. Problems with a 'target' approach to access in primary care: a qualitative study. *British Journal of General Practice* 2004;**54**:364–6.
3. Eisner M and Britten N. What do general practice receptionists think and feel about their work? *British Journal of General Practice* 1999;**49**:103–6.
4. Gallagher M, Pearson P, Drinkwater C and Guy J. Managing patient demand: a qualitative study of appointment making in general practice. *British Journal of General Practice* 2001;**51**:280–5.
5. Arber S and Sawyer L. The role of the receptionist in general practice: a 'dragon behind the desk'? *Social Science and Medicine* 1985;**20**:911–21.
6. Dixon C, Tompkins C, Allgar V and Wright N. Abusive behaviour experienced by primary care receptionists: a cross-sectional survey. *Family Practice* 2004;**21**:137–9.
7. Pascoe S, Neal R and Allgar V. Open-access versus bookable appointment systems: survey of patients attending appointments with general practitioners. *British Journal of General Practice* 2004;**54**:367–9.
8. Oldham J. *Advanced Access in Primary Care*. Manchester: National Primary Care Development Team, 2001.
9. Womack J, Jones D and Roos D. *The Machine That Changed the World: The story of lean production*. New York: Rawson, 1990.
10. Salisbury C. Does Advanced Access work for patients and practices? *British Journal of General Practice* 2004;**54**:330–1.
11. Department of Health. *The NHS Plan*. London: Department of Health, 2002.
12. www.bma.org.uk/ap.nsf/Content/news4nov06 [accessed November 2006].
13. Hildebrandt D, Westfall J and Smith P. After-hours telephone triage affects patient safety. *Journal of Family Practice* 2003;**52**:222–7.
14. NHS careers. *Emergency Medical Dispatcher/Patient Transport Services Call Handler*. www.nhs24.com/html/content/default.asp?page=s3_1 [accessed November 2006]. 2004.
15. NHS 24. *Vacancies – Call handler*. www.nhs24.com/default.asp?page=s3_1 [accessed November 2006]. 2004.
16. AMSPAR. *The AMSPAR Receptionist Programme and Certificate in General Practice Reception*. www.amspar.com/cgpr.php [accessed November 2006]. 2005.
17. Robbins M. *Medical Receptionists and Secretaries Handbook*. Oxford: Radcliffe, 2002.

CHAPTER 6

The role of the primary care nurse in telephone consultations

It is difficult to separate the role of senior practice nursing staff in telephone consultations from their roles in chronic disease management and/or minor illness management, since both require the use of a sound clinical knowledge base and communication and management skills. Primary care nursing roles have expanded and adapted as more and varied tasks have become incorporated into the services delivered in the community.[1,2] Nurse-initiated telephone consultations are an effective and efficient way of following up patients with chronic disease[3,4] or who are being supported through lifestyle changes such as smoking cessation.[5] Home visit requests can be managed by initial assessment by a practice nurse; in a study from Gateshead (UK) more than half of patients were appropriately directed to surgery consultations or telephone advice.[6] Nurses are generally positive about having telephone queries from patients put through to them.[7] This chapter will focus on the triage function, which requires a complex set of communication, decision-making and advice-giving skills as well as clinical knowledge.

Safety of nurse triage

In a study of quality monitoring of nurse telephone triage Richards *et al.* listened to audiotapes of 216 triage calls made by eight nurses at the three surgery sites of a large practice in York (UK).[8] The calls lasted between one and 11 minutes, the median duration being three minutes. There were seven triage options to choose from:

- telephone advice only
- telephone consultation with GP
- same-day appointment with triage nurse
- same-day appointment with GP
- home visit from GP
- routine nurse appointment
- routine GP appointment.

Tapes were assessed according to the breadth and depth of information sought and the appropriateness of the triage decision. Thirty-eight per cent of calls were managed without the need for GP involvement on the same day. Seven calls were assessed as 'potentially dangerous' triage outcomes. Five of these involved children and the calls were criticised for not containing sufficient information about level of dehydration (in a five-month-old with a gastrointestinal upset) or to exclude meningococcal disease.

The management decisions in a similar number of telephone calls conducted by nurses in a health centre in Sweden,[9] where nurse triage is commonplace, were compared with decisions made in subsequent face-to-face consultations with both the original nurse and a GP. Only 4 per cent of patients had their diagnosis changed after seeing the nurse and 1 per cent after seeing the doctor. There were no 'near misses' although patients who were considered to be seriously ill and advised to present themselves to hospital were excluded from the study. Patients are highly satisfied with the Swedish system and half of calls are managed with self-care advice.[10] Timpka and Arborelius[11] described how complex the nurse triage task is: two-thirds of 31 telephone consultations conducted by five nurses at a Swedish health centre presented dilemmas in terms of management decision-making and one-third caused difficulty because of the nurses' mistrust of the patient's account of the clinical problem. A questionnaire study identified decision-making as one of the three most frequent concerns of telephone nurses, alongside lack of resources and third-party consultations.[12]

A study from New Zealand assessed the triage decisions of nurses blind to the fact that the calls under scrutiny were being made by simulated patients.[13] This 'mystery shopper' methodology revealed a wide discrepancy between expected and actual triage outcomes of four different clinical scenarios: a man with a past history of rheumatic fever presenting with a sore throat; a woman with risk factors for thromboembolic disease calling with chest pain; a woman with genitourinary symptoms; and the mother of a sick child. The authors expected the triage nurses to refer all the callers for further medical assessment but this occurred only half of the time.

Signposting the triage function

The involvement of nurses in the management of demand for same-day appointments may be new for some patients, so an explanation of the role of the triage nurse may be helpful in order that the patient understands that his or her problem is being handled by the practice team and not necessarily the GP. Potential statements that might fulfil this purpose are:

good morning Mister Matthews this is Pat one of the practice nurses ringing back about Margaret

oh yes

I'm working with Doctor Black (1.0) we're both on duty for urgent problems today.

AND: I'd like to find out a bit more about the problem because sometimes we can give advice over the phone

OR: I need to ask you a few questions to work out what kind of treatment will help

During the remainder of the consultation the nurse aims to gather sufficient information to make a safe triage decision.

Decision-making

Nurses and nurse practitioners are as much 'in the dark' as any clinician when it comes to the relatively cueless environment of the telephone consultation and every triage decision made by telephone carries with it a degree of risk. Evidence from interviews with nurses shows that they compensate by visualising their patients, building up pictures in their mind's eye of the predicaments being presented to them.[14,15] In keeping with the clinical reasoning strategies adopted by experts such pictures can be compared with previously experienced patterns of illness.[16] The cognitive strategies used by nurses in their assessments of patients are similar to those used by doctors in diagnosis, although the emphasis in the nursing process is on the patient's condition or situation rather than the biomedical problem.[17] Symptoms and signs that represent 'red flags' or significant risk can be managed by further face-to-face assessment. Checklists of closed questions, such as when a parent mentions a rash in the context of an acute febrile illness, can be used to help nurses minimise the risks:

hello?

hello it's Pat here one of the nurses ringing back about Heidi.

thank you I don't know if I need to bring her in but she's been poorly for two days now.

well let's see if we can work it out could you tell me what's been happening from when it started?

just the temperature really and she's just not interested in anything

temperature and not interested ok

she was perfectly alright Sunday for her party now all she wants to do is flop on the sofa

she had a birthday? how old is she now.

two.

ok so I'm picturing Heidi flopping on the sofa with a temperature for two days.

yeah oh and there's this rash too?

tell me about that.

small red spots mostly on her tummy and chest you can't feel them or anything

> Nurse adopts a collaborative approach from the outset

> Nurse repeats mother's phrase as a signal for her to go on

> She summarises the predicament using visualisation, which acts as a prompt for more information

you mean they're flat?

yeah

and definitely red

bright red

I usually get mums and dads to say as much as they can about rashes because some are more serious than others.

well it did cross my mind.

what did.

meningitis.

you're right to be concerned let's test the rash do you have a glass?

I pressed one on earlier and it seemed to go away.

well done and are there any new spots since we have been talking.

funny you should say that I think one's just come on her leg,

shall we get the doctor to see Heidi just to make sure.

I'd be happier if he did see her.

ok

> She uses a neutral statement to elicit mother's (and perhaps revealing her own) concerns about the rash

> Nurse offers a face-to-face consultation in response to the concerns and uncertainty

Safe advice-giving

When nurses make a triage decision to give telephone advice to patients and carers, it is good practice to describe worsening symptoms and leave the caller with a plan of what to do should the clinical situation deteriorate. Other safety net strategies include making a return call later in the day, providing callers with the telephone number for the out-of-hours service and advising patients who live alone to ask a friend or relative to visit or stay overnight.

Charles Wilson

morning Mister Wilson Pat the nurse speaking

oh yes the receptionist said you'd be calling is this a new system?

that's right Mister Wilson I call patients back and help decide who needs to come today as we don't have enough appointments for everyone.

> Nurse explains her triage function

well shall I describe my symptoms?

please do.

ok it's right big toe excruciating pain came on last night never had anything like it before can't walk on it now red and swollen wife thinks it's the gout.

it could well be how do you feel in yourself?

tired.

oh dear I'm guessing you didn't get much sleep [last night

[tried

paracetamol and something the wife got for her back (0.5) co-codamol neither did much good.

I'm sorry let me ask about the toe which part is swollen.

where it joins the foot.

and how far does the redness go.

not far perhaps half an inch in all directions.

I see and is it hot to the touch?

burning.

well I'm inclined to agree with your wife about her diagnosis of gout

so what can I take?

there's another type of painkiller that's anti-inflammatory like aspirin

she could go to the chemist for me.

it should be ok for you as long as you're not allergic have asthma or any indigestion problems

none of the above

can she pick up a prescription from here on the way?

yes.

I'll ask the doctor to print off a prescription for some tablets they should start working today but if you're no better by tomorrow please call back.

I certainly will thanks for your help.

no problem goodbye.

> Nurse attempts to address the illness experience and express empathy

> A series of closed questions to narrow down the diagnostic possibilities

> Nurse makes a treatment decision and anticipates approval by her medical colleague; this does not constitute nurse prescribing

Protocols

Practice nurses and nurse practitioners are responsible for their own acts and omissions, are regulated by and can be insured through their professional body, the Royal College of Nursing. Some practices indemnify their employed nurses through group insurance schemes provided by the medical defence bodies. As the role of the primary care nurse has expanded so has his or her professional autonomy. Nurses not only undertake work that is traditionally delegated by medical colleagues (health promotion and disease prevention activities), but also new work arising from professional development such as smoking cessation. The broader the role, the greater the need for medico-legal protection, and protocols can help nurses practise within agreed boundaries[18] in keeping with their level of training, in recognition of their autonomy and to legitimise their knowledge.[19]

Decision-support software

The use of computer programs to guide nursing staff through triage and advice-giving by telephone was referred to in Chapter 1. Telephone Advice System (TAS © the Plain Software Company) was developed as a response to the needs expressed by staff working in a London accident and emergency (A&E) department.[20] The same team described its successful implementation in both A&E and general practice through a training programme.[21] It is used by many GP co-operatives and some individual practices.

TAS allows the triage nurse to open sets of questions in response to each symptom the patient presents.[22] The program allocates a colour code to the patient's potential answers according to their clinical significance. The colours range from red, indicating immediate referral is necessary, to blue, meaning self-care advice is appropriate. For example a patient calling about abdominal pain and vomiting may be asked two sets of questions. Replies to questions about abdominal pain (site, severity, speed of onset, whether constant or colicky, etc.) may generate coloured flags of moderate urgency but if the patient confesses to having vomited blood in the 'vomiting' pathway, the level of urgency jumps to red. The software generates the coloured hierarchy of triage decisions by allocating predetermined scores to the symptoms as they are recorded by the nurse.

Dale, Crouch and Lloyd described the use of TAS in British primary care.[23] Over a six-month period in the autumn and winter of 1996–7, 25 practice nurses handled over 10,000 calls. The mean call duration was 6.73 minutes, and the mean number of question sets per call was 3 (a total of 111 were used altogether). There were roughly equal numbers of patient triaged to be seen face-to-face the same day, either in primary care or A&E, as were given advice. The researchers observed a two-fold variation in triage decisions between nurses: some gave home care advice to 65 per cent of callers while at the other extreme this rate was 35 per cent. This variation illustrates the function of the program as an adjunct to clinical judgement. In the words of the Plain Software Company:

> Instead of the traditional approach of using binary algorithms for clinical decision support, our software is based upon a patient–centred model that supports health care professionals' judgment and expertise through enhancing normal consultation processes. This increases the safety and efficacy of consultation through facilitation, rather than imposition.[24]

NHS Direct, the 24-hour nurse-led telephone and internet-based information and triage service added to the NHS in 1998, has piloted several computer programs. Until 2001, three software systems were in use: TAS, Personal Health Adviser (© McKesson HBOC) and Centramax (© McKesson HBOC). During 2001 a fourth, the NHS Clinical Assessment System (CAS © AXA Assistance), was implemented as the national standard system across all sites in England and Wales.

These systems were compared by presenting cases based on low–priority 999 calls to nurses in four NHS Direct centres.[25] The summary statistic derived from the data (kappa) was 0.375, indicating low to moderate agreement between the systems. The sensitivity and specificity of each system was determined by comparing each soft-ware-supported triage decision with data collected by the ambulance crews and the hospitals to which the patients were conveyed, each having been coded as 'necessary' (75 per cent of cases) or 'unnecessary' (25 per cent) visits to A&E. TAS and Centramax had high sensitivity (70 per cent and 78 per cent respectively) but low specificity (33 per cent for both) while Personal Health Adviser and CAS had low sensitivity (51 per cent and 49 per cent) but higher specificity (52 per cent and 59 per cent respectively).

CAS is based on 180 symptom–based algorithms (www.casservicesltd.com/). The prompts that are provided for the nurse are responsive to the age and gender of the caller, and include questions intended to identify serious pathology if it exists. 'Disposition override switches' allow the nurse to use clinical judgement but an ulti-mate triage decision must be made for each caller: home treatment advice; urgent or routine appointment with a GP; or emergency attendance at an A&E department.

The top ten symptoms presented to NHS Direct nurses are:[26]
• fever
• abdominal pain
• vomiting
• rash
• cough
• diarrhoea
• headache
• cold and flu
• toothache
• chest pain.

Twenty–four nurses at 12 NHS Direct sites were interviewed about their roles and that of the software they use.[27] Nurses reported that decision–support software was an essential safety net for themselves and their patients, enabled them to be consistent in the advice they gave, provided information about unfamiliar prob-lems and helped to structure their consultations. Nurses regarded themselves as autonomous in the decision–making process, overriding the programme when the clinical context doesn't fit with the computer's recommendations. Nurse and soft-ware appeared to function as an integrated system.

The relative effects of practice nurse and NHS Direct telephone triage of daytime calls to primary care were reported from York (UK).[28] NHS Direct nurses took 6.9 minutes longer than practice nurses to triage their share of the 4700 randomised patients. NHS Direct triage was more likely to lead to a same–day appointment with a GP and 50 additional appointments were required over the six–month duration of the study.

No difference was detected between the two groups of patients in terms of consulting behaviour in the month following their calls. Costs were estimated to be £2.88 greater per patient in NHS Direct triage group, which related to nursing staff costs.

Hagan *et al.* evaluated Info-Santé, the equivalent service in Québec, Canada, and found that it saved money for the health economy in the province.[29] Info-Santé was introduced in the mid-1980s to ease the burden on A&E departments. Its nurses helped to develop computerised protocols in 1995. In a 1997 survey, 4700 callers expressed considerable satisfaction with the quality of the service. Responders to the survey estimated that the service saved them an average of five hours of time and half would have attended A&E had Info-Santé not been available.

Personal development

Educational needs will depend on the practice or out-of-hours service context and the extent to which telephone medicine is to be developed by the whole team. Professional development in this area therefore should be coordinated with that of other health professional and reception staff. Nurses may wish to investigate training opportunities in minor illness diagnosis and management such as that provided by the Minor Illness Beacon.[30] This nurse-led resource is based in a practice in Luton (UK). A team responsible for demonstrating the effectiveness of minor illness management by practice nurses[31] designed a university-accredited training course involving one day's study per week for three months. Universities known to offer opportunities for postgraduate nursing study relevant to telephone consultation (all accessed July 2006) are:

- King's College London School of Medicine, Department of General Practice and Primary Care, http://gppc.kcl.ac.uk
- Bournemouth, Institute of Health and Community Studies, www.bournemouth.ac.uk/ihcs/index.html
- University of Greenwich, School of Health and Social Care, www.gre.ac.uk/schools/health/index.htm
- University of Stirling, Department of Nursing and Midwifery, www.nm.stir.ac.uk/
- Homerton School of Health Studies, Cambridge, www.health-homerton.ac.uk/
- University of Central Lancashire, Faculty of Health, www.uclan.ac.uk/facs/health/index.htm.

Practical application

Nurses and nurse practitioners respond positively to being given the responsibility for triaging and advising patients by telephone. Patients are satisfied with such a service and its safety can be enhanced by the use of protocols and decision-support software. Nurse-led telephone consultations should be included in a practice or out-of-hours service as part of a system to make the most efficient and cost-effective use of the skills among the clinical team. Guidance for nurses and their employing organisations is offered in Box 6.1 below.

> ## Box 6.1 Guidance on the role of nursing staff in telephone consultations
>
> ### Triage
>
> Primary care nurses can adapt their assessment skills to formulate diagnoses and make triage decisions.
>
> With further training nurses can appropriately manage up to half of calls from patients requesting home visits or same-day appointments with doctors.
>
> Patients are satisfied with the telephone advice they receive from nurses.
>
> ### Policies and protocols
>
> Nurses should be familiar with practice or out-of-hours service policies on home-visiting criteria, prescribing and referrals.
>
> They should be aware of the obligations of the practice's GMS contract or the out-of-hours service's National Quality Requirements.
>
> Structured questions or lists of points to cover are helpful to improve safety and effectiveness.
>
> Protocols facilitate chronic disease management and health promotion activities conducted by nurses.
>
> ### Decision-support tools
>
> The use of decision-support software doubles the length of telephone consultations.
>
> Nurses feel more confident and empowered with such tools.
>
> Clinical judgement can still be exercised.

Exercises

The exercises that follow enable readers involved in clinical management to review and reflect on recent cases from their own practice. Patient satisfaction is difficult to elicit reliably without a validated instrument, preferably administered by an impartial observer, but the clinician may learn something about his or her performance by making direct follow-up contact with patients.

Exercise 11

Objective: to use outcome data from telephone consultations to identify unmet patient needs and personal development needs.

During your next session of telephone assessments, keep a record of a sample of patients and carers with whom you consulted. Choose some from each of the triage outcomes: direct admission, home visit, face-to-face consultation at surgery and telephone advice. Ask permission from each caller to follow the situation up and track the outcome of your calls.

- How satisfied were the callers with the advice you gave?
- How many of your diagnoses were correct?
- How many patients attended for follow-up as instructed?
- How many subsequently consulted one of your colleagues for another opinion?

Exercise 12

Objective: to use outcome data from an out-of-hours provider to identify strengths and weaknesses in its service.

Examine a week's worth of out-of-hours contacts between your patients and the out-of-hours service that took place one month ago. Consider feeding back your findings to the service.

- How would you rate the quality of the communication?
- How would you rate the appropriateness of the clinical care?
- What proportion of triage decisions were incorrect in retrospect?
- How many patients presented again within 14 days and why?

References

1. Lorentzon M and Hooker J. Nurse practitioners, practice nurses and nurse specialists: what's in a name? (editorial). *Journal of Advanced Nursing* 1996;**24**:649–51.
2. Atkin K and Lunt N. Negotiating the role of the practice nurse in general practice. *Journal of Advanced Nursing* 1996;**24**:498–505.
3. Pinnock H, Bawden R, Proctor S, Wolfe S, Scullion J, Price D, *et al.* Accessibility, acceptability, and effectiveness in primary care of routine telephone review of asthma: pragmatic, randomised controlled trial. *British Medical Journal* 2003;**326**:477–9.
4. Kim H and Oh J. Adherence to diabetes control recommendations: impact of nurse telephone calls. *Journal of Advanced Nursing* 2003;**44**:256–61.
5. Stead L, Lancaster T and Perera R. Telephone counselling for smoking cessation (Cochrane Review). *The Cochrane Library, Issue 4*. Chichester, UK: John Wiley and Sons Ltd, 2004.
6. Jones K, Gilbert P, Little J and Wilkinson K. Nurse triage for house call requests in a Tyneside general practice: patients' views and effect on doctor workload. *British Journal of General Practice* 1998;**48**:1303–6.
7. Williams S, Crouch R and Dale J. Providing health-care advice by telephone. *Professional Nurse* 1995;**10**:750–2.
8. Richards D, Meakins J, Tawfik J, Godfrey L, Dutton E and Heywood P. Quality monitoring of nurse telephone triage: pilot study. *Journal of Advanced Nursing* 2004;**47**:551–60.
9. Marklund B, Koritz P, Bjorkander E and Bengtsson C. How well do nurse-run telephone consultations and consultations in the surgery agree? Experience in Swedish primary health care. *British Journal of General Practice* 1991;**41**:462–5.
10. Wahlberg A and Wredling R. Telephone nursing: calls and caller satisfaction. *International Journal of Nursing Practice* 1999;**5**:164.
11. Timpka T and Arborelius E. The primary-care nurse's dilemmas: a study of knowledge use and need during telephone consultations. *Journal of Advanced Nursing* 1990;**15**:1457–65.
12. Wahlberg A, Cedersund E and Wredling R. Telephone nurses' experience of problems with telephone advice in Sweden. *Journal of Clinical Nursing* 2003;**12**:37.
13. Moriarty H, McLeod D and Dowell A. Mystery shopping in health service evaluation. *British Journal of General Practice* 2003;**53**:942–6.
14. Pettinari C and Jessop L. 'Your ears become your eyes': managing the absence of visibility in NHS Direct. *Journal of Advanced Nursing* 2001;**36**:668–75.

15. Edwards B. Seeing is believing – picture building: a key component of telephone triage. *Journal of Clinical Nursing* 1998;**7**:51–8.
16. Sackett DL, Haynes RB, Guyatt GH and Tugwell P. *Clinical Epidemiology. A basic science for clinical medicine.* Boston: Little Brown, 1991.
17. Crow R, Chase J and Lamond D. The cognitive component of nursing assessment: an analysis. *Journal of Advanced Nursing* 1995;**22**:206–12.
18. Pennels C. Nurse prescribing. Protocols for safety. *Nursing Times* 1999;**95**:12–13.
19. Manias E and Street A. Legitimation of nurses' knowledge through policies and protocols in clinical practice. *Journal of Advanced Nursing* 2000;**32**:1467–75.
20. Dale J, Williams S and Crouch R. Development of telephone advice in A&E: establishing the views of staff. *Nursing Standard* 1995;**9**:28–31.
21. Crouch R, Woodfield H, Dale J and Patel A. Telephone assessment and advice: a training programme. *Nursing Standard* 1997;**11**:41–4.
22. The Plain Software Company Ltd. *Assessing Patients Using TAS Odyssey.* www.plain.co.uk/PDF/TAS2.pdf [accessed November 2006]. 2004.
23. Dale J, Crouch R and Lloyd D. Primary care: nurse-led telephone triage and advice out-of-hours. *Nursing Standard* 1998;**12**:41–5.
24. The Plain Software Company Ltd. *The Company: Our approach.* www.plain.co.uk/company.htm [accessed November 2005]. 2004.
25. O'Cathain A, Webber E, Nicholl J, Munro J and Knowles E. NHS Direct: consistency of triage outcomes. *Emergency Medicine Journal* 2003;**20**:289–92.
26. NHS Direct. *NHS Direct Four Years On.* 2002.
27. O'Cathain A, Sampson F, Munro J, Thomas K and Nicholl J. Nurses' views of using computerized decision support software in NHS Direct. *Journal of Advanced Nursing* 2004;**45**:280–6.
28. Richards D, Godfrey L, Tawfik J, Ryan M, Meakins J, Dutton E, *et al.* NHS Direct versus general practice based triage for same day appointments in primary care: cluster randomised controlled trial. *British Medical Journal* 2004;**329**:774–7.
29. Hagan L, Morin D and Lepine R. Evaluation of telenursing outcomes: satisfaction, self-care practices, and cost savings. *Public Health Nursing* 2000;**17**:305–13.
30. Minor Illness Beacon. *Minor Illness Courses.* www.minorillness.co.uk/min/services/courses.htm [accessed November 2006]. 2004.
31. Shum C, Humphreys A, Wheeler D, Cochrane M-A, Skoda S and Clement S. Nurse management of patients with minor illnesses in general practice; multicentre, randomised controlled trial. *British Medical Journal* 2000;**320**:1038–43.

CHAPTER 7

The role of the GP in telephone consultations

Whether single-handed or in partnership, in daytime or out-of-hours work, GPs are responsible for managing their workload and delegating tasks to their employed and attached staff. The previous two chapters have demonstrated that other primary care team members can develop skills and take a share of administrative (receptionists and call handlers) and clinical (nurses and nurse practitioners) responsibilities.

The evidence on the effectiveness of GP telephone consultations on overall daytime workload is mixed. Such a service provides an alternative form of contact for patients who already make regular use of the practice[1,2] and can reduce demand for same-day appointments,[3] but the time spent on the telephone may exceed the time gained by saving a face-to-face consultation.[4,5] Increasing the number of outgoing telephone calls incurs significant costs to a practice[3] but telephone follow-up of chronic disease can benefit the local health economy.[6] A study in Cumbria (UK), intended to discover what proportion of daytime face-to-face consultations could be managed by telephone, demonstrated only 5.5 per cent agreement between doctors and patients in a sample of 1067 consultations.[7] Therefore it was not possible to predict which problems were suitable for telephone management. This may explain the lack of efficiency in telephone medicine as far as the practice is concerned, but patients value the opportunity to access primary care by telephone.[8]

In the context of demand management and access targets,[9] alternatives to the face-to-face consultation have their place in the repertoire of services a practice can offer. The patient's agenda may be apparent prior to the call or may emerge during it. The medium of the telephone may facilitate or inhibit the expression of the agenda: the relative anonymity afforded by speech-only communication may allow patients to reveal personal problems, but the businesslike interaction may limit the content to biomedical symptoms. The GP must therefore be as prepared for any eventuality in telephone consultation as he or she is for face-to-face encounters, including the termination of a call when patient circumstances dictate that a telephone encounter should be converted to a face-to-face appointment.

Daytime telephone consultations can serve a variety of purposes:

- in clinical management
  - assessing a new clinical problem for triage, e.g. a request for a home visit
  - offering a second opinion or taking over management from a colleague
  - giving advice when uncertainty is manageable, e.g. to well-known patients
  - multi-tasking, e.g. conducting a surgery while on call for emergencies
  - following up a clinical problem, e.g. checking adherence to treatment
  - discussing patients with colleagues or making referrals to secondary care
- in practice organisation
  - arranging the issue of a repeat prescription or medical certificate
  - giving the results of investigations
  - fielding a complaint or occasionally a compliment
  - speaking to third parties about a patient, e.g. relatives, neighbours, social workers and the police.

Out-of-hours consultations are almost entirely telephone-mediated in the first instance, with face-to-face contact as an alternative or additional service provided after telephone assessment. The functions of the out-of-hours telephone consultation are two-fold: reaching a shared triage decision about a clinical problem; and giving advice if that decision does not entail a subsequent face-to-face consultation. Caller satisfaction with GP telephone consultation out-of-hours was found to be low in an interview study of 47 patients and carers who had contacted an inner-city GP-led cooperative in the preceding seven to ten days.[10] Common reasons for patient dissatisfaction were the issue of trusting a telephone diagnosis without a physical examination, being made to feel that the doctor's time was being wasted, anxiety about describing symptoms over the phone, and understanding and following advice. Therefore high-quality and well-rehearsed communication skills are especially important in the out-of-hours period, when GPs are more frequently required to:

- negotiate with patients and carers about the need for and location of a face-to-face consultation
- deal with their own emotional state and the expressed emotions of the caller
- avoid conflict, particularly in the area of home visit requests
- establish degree of departure from the usual state of patients with chronic problems.

This chapter uses excerpts from fictitious GP telephone consultations, in daytime practice and out-of-hours, to illustrate some of the common functions and skills listed above, each preceded by further theory. The first continues the scenario about a gentleman with suspected gout from Chapter 6.

The second opinion

GPs engaged in telephone triage may be asked to conduct a consultation with a patient or carer who has already spoken to a nurse or other professional colleague. The reason for the transfer from one clinician to another should be communicated clearly before the second contact is made. The following are possible reasons:

- the first clinician is unsure what triage decision to make
- he or she wishes the doctor to reinforce advice already given
- the patient has insisted on speaking to the doctor.

Supporting a colleague helps with the cohesion of the clinical team and presents a consistent approach to patients and carers:

seven seven oh three four nine?

morning Missus Wilson it's Doctor Black

I'm sorry to bother you it's just that Charles has this bad foot and all that's happened is nurse has told him to send me up there for a prescription but he can't take any weight on it.

Caller expresses dissatisfaction with initial nurse triage

what concerns you the most.

well you know it's the golf club dinner tonight and I have no idea how he's going to get there can't you pop in?

I'm sorry but I can't justify a home visit based on the information we have Missus Wilson.

Underlying concern elicited allowing GP to explain practice visiting policy

but surely you need to see things to know what to do.

actually I don't most of the time and a lot of problems can be dealt with by nurses just as well as by doctors.

well I don't know=

=I've read Pat's notes and it looks like a pretty good description of a gout attack to me.

it's been a few years since I was nursing but we didn't make diagnoses in those days.

well the role of the practice nurse has changed a lot I would have recommended the same myself,

GP supports colleague's triage decision and gives further explanation of the expanded role of the nurse

really?

tell Charles to take three of the tablets straight away then one every eight hours after that preferably with or after food let me know if he gets any indigestion with the medication but he'll notice the difference by this time tomorrow.

alright doctor,

and I'll phone him at the end of the week.

ok I'll tell him.

Familiarity with the patient

Knowing a patient can be extremely useful in the telephone management of new problems or acute exacerbations of chronic problems. Familiarity with patients' histories, illness behaviour and social circumstances is one of the strengths of general practice: such knowledge helps to build the doctor–patient relationship over time and reduces uncertainty in both communication and diagnosis. This is particularly relevant in people with mental health problems, personality disorders or medically unexplained symptoms. The following represents the opening seconds of a consultation with a young man with chronic anxiety and a history of deliberate self-harm:

hello?

hello Kevin it's Doctor White speaking.

hi doc it's my heart again,

your heart.

yeah been thumping and fluttering all day=

=oh dear=

=off and on

I see anything else

just the usual ache and I'm knackered

anything else happening at the moment?

no I'm on my own Tracey went into hysterics earlier and walked out

what happened?

she's just touchy at this time of the month.

how did it make you feel,

pretty cheesed off to be honest nearly took some tablets.

but you didn't.

wish I did then all this heart business wouldn't have come back

ok let's think about how to handle this Kevin have you got a few more minutes?

> Patient refers to previous consultations about palpitations

> Doctor elicits trigger for Kevin's physical symptoms . . .

> . . . and explores the possible behavioural consequences

Multi-tasking

The on-call doctor may have to field additional telephone calls in order to triage visit requests or urgent problems arising between surgeries. Having to be in two places simultaneously is a common cause of stress for the on-call doctor. Conflicting commitments may influence the decisions made, such as putting off a home visit until after a meeting or referring a patient to hospital on the basis of a telephone history alone. An elderly woman has fallen down at home and her husband calls to request an urgent home visit. These are the closing exchanges of the initial consultation:

ok so she's at the bottom of the stairs and the pain's mostly in her hip and you can't move her.

that's right doctor she's sitting up now but I don't like the look of this leg.

well look it's nearly half past three and I'm starting a surgery here how about if we just get her into hospital and let them x-ray her hip.

shall I call the ambulance?

yes please and I'll fax a letter over there.

The next telephone call is conducted with little preparation:

Doctor Jones orthopaedics.

good afternoon sorry to trouble you but I wonder if you would have a look at a seventy five year old woman who fell downstairs just now and may have a fractured neck of femur.

I don't see why not which side has she injured?

right no left actually I'm not sure I only spoke to her husband

oh you haven't examined her?

no I'm afraid I have a waiting room that's starting to fill up

not as full as casualty at the moment ok what's her name?

A better outcome can be achieved by presenting the relevant information concisely as follows:

Doctor Jones orthopaedics.

hello there it's Doctor Green from High Street Surgery I'd appreciate some help with a patient who I haven't seen because surgery is starting in a couple of minutes but the history is pretty convincing for a fractured neck of femur.

right.

Doris Greaves is a seventy five year old usually fit and well lives with her husband she fell down the last three stairs onto her left hip can't weight bear and the lower limb is shortened and externally rotated according to the husband's description.

ok can you send her to casualty?

she'll be on the way shortly thanks.

Interruptions

Telephone interruptions during a face-to-face consultation are occasional inconveniences with which the GP has to cope. Receptionists find having to interrupt consulting doctors stressful and have a high threshold for doing so. Behaviour under these conditions may affect the caller on hold, the patient in the consulting room, the receptionist and the GP. Frustration expressed verbally and non-verbally can affect working relationships so it is important to separate roles from personalities. GPs should have a planned response to interruptions to include the following:

- breaking off from a face-to-face consultation
- receiving the urgent message
- making a rapid assessment in order to prioritise
- abandoning or resuming the face-to-face consultation.

When a consultation is interrupted the patient needs to be put safely 'on hold' with an explanation that an urgent call has come through. Some doctors ask the patient to leave the consulting room, while others leave the patient and take the call elsewhere. Patients who are undressed or distressed should probably stay where they are. Any sense of frustration should be guarded against before lifting the receiver and care taken to avoid undue influence by any competing commitments. Dr Green thought that his patient with the suspected femoral neck fracture was safely on her way to hospital. The receptionist receives a call that necessitates an interruption:

sorry doctor but I think you had better speak to this gentleman it's about Missus Greaves.

ok thanks hello Doctor Green here.

afternoon doc Joe Simpkins here paramedic.

oh.

yeah we've responded to a nines call to your patient Doris Greaves I believe you spoke to the husband earlier.

that's right she fell downstairs and has probably broken her hip

it looks like it we've assessed her and the pulse is eighty regular BP one sixty ninety alert and orientated we've given her some entonox but now she doesn't want to go in the ambulance.

why not?

something about the hospital and a neighbour who died there last week

I see can I speak to her briefly? I'm in the middle of surgery so I haven't got long

ok doc here she is

A few minutes spent on dealing with the urgent problem adequately should enable the GP to refocus on the patient in the surgery safe in the knowledge that he or she can continue the consultation. When doctor and patient are reunited a brief apology and explanation are usually readily accepted. If the consultation has to be abandoned it pays to make arrangements to see or speak to the patient at a later date and to involve reception staff in facilitating this as well as asking them to explain to other patients in the waiting room that their GP has had to go out on an urgent visit.

Follow-up

The telephone can be used proactively to communicate with patients about their ongoing symptoms and adherence to, or effect of, treatment. Although this can be delegated to other members of the primary care team, the GP may wish to make personal contact for various reasons:

- a diagnosis has not yet been made and the passage of time is being used to test hypotheses
- the doctor has a special clinical interest in the patient's problem
- the doctor is the most appropriate 'key worker' for the particular patient
- telephone follow-up as a substitute for a home visit or an interim form of contact between planned surgery attendances[6]
- the doctor is conducting an audit or research project.[11]

Investigation results

The communication of both normal and abnormal investigations to patients requires a safe and reliable system. The common policy of 'no news is good news' has been shown to be less than satisfactory in an accident and emergency department in Boston (USA), the staff of which took throat swabs from patients attending with sore throats.[12] Errors in the communication of results can lead to a delay in diagnosis with medico-legal consequences for the physician.[13] One-hundred-and-sixty-eight primary care doctors in the Boston area reported spending a mean of 74 minutes per day on managing test results but less than half were satisfied with the systems they used.[14]

The patient can use the telephone to contact the practice for his or her results. Some practices set up a dedicated telephone line for such queries or a specific time of day when an appropriate member of staff is available to answer the calls. Alternatively the clinicians in the practice who order the tests can take the responsibility of communicating the results to the patient, whether normal or abnormal, and this can be done efficiently by telephone. There is a confidentiality issue, however, when a third party or answering machine is reached instead of the intended patient. Under these circumstances it is best to leave a message asking the patient to contact the surgery.

Negotiation

Patients who perceive difficulty in accessing their own practice may use out-of-hours services inappropriately and GPs fielding these calls face the challenge of negotiating a more reasonable plan:

hello there Doctor Brown speaking.

oh yes hello it's about my little boy I've been worried about him all day.

all day.

yes he woke up with a temperature so I kept him off school,

yes?

he complained of a sore throat and a headache so I gave him some paracetamol=

=right=

=suspension which helped for a couple of hours but since lunchtime he's just been miserable.

why didn't you contact your own surgery during the day?

oh you can never get an appointment with them they're so busy.

If the subsequent history is consistent with the early stages of an upper respiratory tract infection with no worrying clinical features this consultation could continue with:

so from what you've told me I think Charlie has a throat infection that is making his ear hurt and the temperature is giving him the headache and I'm sorry he's so miserable with it.

he is really miserable.

what you have been doing so far today is absolutely correct and I think he'll be due for another dose of paracetamol in another hour.

ok.

the other thing that would help him is a bit more to drink.

I'll try.

well done and if it turns out to be a bad night or you are still worried in the morning please contact your practice and ask for him to be checked over=

=can't someone do that tonight I'd be much happier,

I'm sorry I can't justify that from what you have told me about him.

but they're always so busy.

I can help by sending a fax telling your own doctor all about Charlie's problems so by the morning they'll be expecting you to make contact if things are still bad.

do you think that will work?

my colleagues send me faxes in the same way and we always try to make room for poorly children.

alright then.

The GP has affirmed the action taken by the anxious mother so far and has used three steps in the negotiation process: a statement about the usual threshold for a face-to-face consultation; advice about what to do should symptoms persist; and an offer to facilitate further care.

Dealing with expressed emotion

Patient and carer anxiety about health problems is heightened in the hours of darkness. Kai conducted a qualitative study in which parents from a disadvantaged inner-city community spoke about their concerns and difficulties in coping with their sick pre-school children.[15,16] Symptoms such as fever and cough, and problems in interpreting signs, worry mothers and fathers, with meningitis being their worst fear. A common example is the young child who wakes with croup:

hello doctor.

yes I got the message about Kylie and your concerns about her breathing

thanks for calling back so quickly we're really panicking here

it must be awful trying to deal with this in the middle of the night tell me what's been happening

well she's had a runny nose for a couple of days and a bit of a cough but nothing like what she's been through the last hour or two

right

the wife's got her sitting on her lap she's making this rasping noise not breathing properly and when you touch oh God she's really burning up doctor

so a bad cough for a couple of hours raspy breathing and she feels really hot to the touch

yes I don't know what to do for her I don't know if she needs to go to hospital she's never been this bad before I nearly called the ambulance I just=

=ok Mister Turpin=

=the wife's crying her eyes out and I'm off work myself with my back God knows what she'd do if I was at work right now=

=ok Mister Turpin it sounds like things are really stressful right now=

=you're telling me doc.

well that's not going to help Kylie she'll get better if things are calmer so let's think this through and see if we can't help Kylie with her breathing and her cough ok?

> Doctor immediately acknowledges parental concerns and makes an empathic statement

> Doctor reflects the symptoms back using neutral rather than emotionally charged speech

> Further empathy in response to the father's sense of panic

> Doctor takes control by focusing on the patient's needs

Conflict avoidance

The technique of agreeing to visit before gathering all the information may appear risky in terms of reinforcing inappropriate help-seeking behaviour on the part of the patient or carer but it can have a remarkable impact on the communication process. Consider a patient in considerable pain calling out-of-hours who believes the only solution to his predicament is an analgesic injection:

hello?

hello it's Doctor Singh speaking.

right now get yourself round here and sort me out.

no problem that's what we're here for now tell me how you got into this state.

> GP 'rolls with the punch' rather than resist the patient's demand

haven't you got my notes?

no your notes are safely locked away at your surgery I'm not from your practice but we look after each other's patients in the evenings.

> GP gives an honest answer and begins to establish a relationship

oh well what do you want to know.

I know that you have back pain and that you are on strong painkillers from your doctor but they're not working tonight.

that's it doctor ooh ah there it goes again I think I need a jab,

tell me exactly where the pain is.

middle low down just below my waistline.

does it spread anywhere from there?

> GP uses that relationship to avoid a response to the next request

no.

and how much can you move your back.

it's completely seized up.

right what about using the toilet any problems?

I can pee alright I haven't tried the other today.

ok Mister Barker I can tell you are in a lot of pain and can't move much but it's a good sign that your bladder works what about your legs any weakness or numbness,

> Important negative features are used to encourage the patient despite his suffering, leaving an opening for negotiation

no nothing like that.

good good so now we need a plan to see you through the night.

so what else can I take?

what have you got in the house?

It is not uncommon in out-of-hours work for there to be a mismatch between the expectations of the patient or carer and that of the clinician taking the call. When the patient expects a face-to-face consultation but the doctor believes this to be unnecessary one or more of the following may be helpful:

- clarify and explore further the patient's underlying concerns
- ask to speak to a relative or carer to obtain a collateral history
- explain the nature of the problem and what the patient should expect, and correct any misunderstandings
- adopt a firm but fair approach for problems that clearly need no attention other than advice during the current out-of-hours period
- refer to policies or evidence, if any are available.

How different from usual?

'Departure from usual state' is a pragmatic strategy in the management of complex patients. A disabled person requiring 24-hour nursing care in a community-based home, bed-bound with cerebral palsy, whose carer calls about a cough and a temperature, may invoke a sense of inevitability in the mind of the triage doctor but a few selected questions may prevent a home visit. This is the second half of a consultation that takes place between a care assistant and a triage GP on duty for an out-of-hours service provider:

so he's managed to take his usual amount of liquidised food and drink, has passed a reasonable amount of urine, managed all his medication and the main concern is his temperature.

> No departure from usual feeding habits and medicine-taking

yes and last time he had a temperature he had more fits than usual.

I can quite understand but the thing with epilepsy is you're more likely to have a fit if your temperature's up even if you've had your medication.

> Doctor acknowledges the carer's concerns then focuses on the main symptom

ok.

let's just think about his chest for a moment you told me it's a dry cough what about his breathing.

his resps are eighteen.

ok that's good and his colour?

> Respiratory rate in normal range and no departure from usual skin colour

about the same as usual.

well I'd be inclined to hang on for the time being as it sounds as though he has a viral infection and is probably quite safe for tonight.

you don't think someone should see him just to cover us?

I know it's your duty to report these things but there's someone here all night so if things change or if you're concerned feel free to ring back.

alright doctor.

Professional development

GPs are responsible for their own continuing professional development within the appraisal and revalidation framework. GP tutors and deaneries will have details of local courses and resources for family doctors who wish to work on their consultation skills. Specific telephone consulting training is offered by the Department of General Practice and Primary Care at King's College London (http://gppc.kcl.ac.uk/guide/ [accessed November 2006]).

Practical application

This chapter has sought to demonstrate the potential of the telephone as an extension of and alternative to the face-to-face consultation for the GP, while acknowledging that the telephone is not likely to reduce the doctor's overall workload. Guidance arising from the many roles of the GP in telephone communication is given in Box 7.1.

Box 7.1 Guidance for GPs in telephone consultation

Calls initiated by patients should be classified according to task and appropriate skills then applied:

- assessment and triage of an acute problem or visit request
- request for information, e.g. of a laboratory test result
- complaint or compliment about the practice or a colleague
- other administrative tasks, e.g. a repeat prescription request.

Calls about patients initiated by third parties should be handled by:

- confirming the identity of the caller
- establishing if patient consent has been given
- acting in the patient's best interest
- recording the communication in the patient's records.

Calls to patients initiated by the GP should be:

- made at a mutually convenient time
- prepared, i.e. all information to hand and management options thought through
- integrated with other patient contacts and with the systems of the primary care team recorded in the patient's records.

Exercises

The following exercises provide opportunities for readers to review and practise the communication skills required for giving information and explaining and planning treatment.

Exercise 13

Objectives: to rehearse and improve upon the communication skills of breaking bad news, explaining abnormal laboratory results and reaching a shared management decision.

You are reviewing laboratory results at the end of evening surgery and notice an unexpected biochemical abnormality on Mark Roberts, a 66-year-old patient who attended earlier in the day with an exacerbation of congestive cardiac failure despite a generous daily dose of a loop diuretic. His renal function had been normal two months ago. You initiated treatment with ramipril and asked the practice nurse to take blood for electrolytes and creatinine. The results are:

- sodium 124 (134–42)
- potassium 5.7 (3.5–4.5)
- creatinine 464 (60–120).

Prepare for a telephone consultation with Mr Roberts by jotting down what you wish to achieve, what the patient's concerns and questions might be, how you will explain the problem and the options for treatment. Try role-playing the consultation with a colleague by sitting back-to-back, each with a (disconnected) telephone handset or mobile telephone.

Exercise 14

Objectives: to achieve a shared clinical decision about anaemia with an unfamiliar patient who may not trust a late evening call from a stranger.

You are on duty for your local out-of-hours service and asked to telephone Mrs Armitage, an 84-year-old woman in a remote village at 9:00 p.m. The initial call was taken by one of the call handlers by a laboratory technician who was obliged to report an abnormal blood test result, the investigation having been arranged by the patient's own GP earlier that day. There is no other clinical information available. The results are:

- white cell count 8.4 (3.9–11.1)
- haemoglobin 4.8 (11.8–14.8)
- platelets 660 (150–350)
- mean red cell volume 63 (76–96).

Plan your telephone call and how you will ensure Mrs Armitage's safety overnight. Consider how you might respond if the patient does not answer the telephone.

References

1. Brown A and Armstrong D. Telephone consultations in general practice: an additional or alternative service? *British Journal of General Practice* 1995;**45**:673–5.
2. Nagle JP, McMahon K, Barbour M and Allen D. Evaluation of the use and usefulness of telephone consultations in one general practice. *British Journal of General Practice* 1992;**42**:190–3.
3. Jiwa M, Mathers N and Campbell M. The effect of GP telephone triage on numbers seeking same-day appointments. *British Journal of General Practice* 2002;**52**:390–1.
4. Richards D, Meakins J, Tawfik J, Godfrey L, Dutton E and Heywood P. Quality monitoring of nurse telephone triage: pilot study. *Journal of Advanced Nursing* 2004;**47**:551–60.
5. Stuart A, Rogers S and Modell M. Evaluation of a direct doctor–patient telephone advice line in general practice. *British Journal of General Practice* 2000;**50**:305–6.
6. Wasson J, Gaudette C, Whaley F, Sauvigne A, Baribeau P and Welch HG. Telephone care as a substitute for routine clinic follow-up. *Journal of the American Medical Association* 1992;**267**:1788–93.
7. Stevenson M, Marsh J and Roderick E. Can patients predict which consultations can be dealt with by telephone? *British Journal of General Practice* 1998;**48**:1772.
8. Hallam L. Access to general practice and general practitioners by telephone: the patient's view. *British Journal of General Practice* 1993;**43**:331–5.
9. Department of Health. *The NHS Plan*. London: Department of Health, 2002.
10. Payne F, Shipman C and Dale J. Patients' experiences of receiving telephone advice from a GP co-operative. *Family Practice* 2001;**18**:156–60.
11. Guthrie R. The effects of postal and telephone reminders on compliance with pravastatin therapy in a national registry: results of the first myocardial infarction risk reduction program. *Clinical Therapeutics* 2001;**23**:970–80.
12. Keren R, Muret-Wagstaff S, Goldmann D and Mandl K. Notifying emergency department patients of negative test results: pitfalls of passive communication. *Pediatric Emergency Care* 2003;**19**:226–30.
13. Bird S. A GP's duty to follow up test results. *Australian Family Physician* 2003;**32**:45–6.
14. Poon E, Gandhi T, Sequist T, Murff H, Karson A and Bates D. 'I wish I had seen this test result earlier!': dissatisfaction with test result management systems in primary care. *Archives of Internal Medicine* 2004;**164**:2223–8.
15. Kai J. What worries parents when their preschool children are acutely ill, and why: a qualitative study. *British Medical Journal* 1996;**313**:983–6.
16. Kai J. Parents' difficulties and information needs in coping with acute illness in preschool children: a qualitative study. *British Medical Journal* 1996;**313**:987–90.

CHAPTER 8

Inter-professional telephone consultations

Effective inter-professional cooperation and communication is vital in contemporary medical practice with its emphasis on multi-disciplinary teamwork and patient-centred care pathways. In a literature review published in 2000, Richards *et al.* described the trend towards the primary care-led NHS with an increasing workload taken on by a more diverse primary healthcare team representing a mix of skills.[1] The authors foresaw the need for integrated, less hierarchical models of team-working as the NHS continues to evolve. There is no single formula for successful multi-disciplinary practice, team-working being culturally and contextually dependent.[2]

Five practices in Dorset (UK) demonstrated improvements in several aspects of their services through inter-professional learning[3] and a team in a Veterans' Affairs medical centre in Oklahoma (USA) introduced a form of telephone triage that allowed patients to be put in touch with a patient service representative, a pharmacist and a nurse, which proved to be a well-received and extremely cost-effective service.[4] An in-house training course for non-medical hospice staff in Bury St Edmunds (UK) helped them better handle stressful incoming telephone calls from patients and relatives.[5]

The preceding chapters in this section have provided examples of how different members of primary care teams in daytime practice and out-of-hours services communicate with patients. This chapter explores the potential of the telephone in facilitating communication between health professionals in daytime practice and in the out-of-hours context, specifically in terms of continuity and sharing of clinical care for patients between GPs and consultants, nurses and paramedics.

Examples of inter-professional telephone communication that might take place during daytime practice are:

- a nurse from a local nursing home calls reception about three patients who are causing concern and merit a visit from the GP
- a community pharmacist leaves a message for a GP about an opioid-dependent patient who has failed to pick up his daily dose of methadone
- a GP calls the local biochemistry lab for advice on what follow-up tests are appropriate for a patient with abnormal liver function tests
- a call from a medical pre-registration house officer to a GP informing her of the imminent discharge of an elderly man who lives alone
- a call from a triage nurse with prescribing skills to a community pharmacist asking him to dispense a course of antibiotics for acute cystitis in a woman who is unable to attend the surgery
- a community midwife contacts the GP on duty requesting a home visit to a woman with acute mastitis.

Telephone consultations between GPs and consultants

Referrals from GPs to hospital consultants have traditionally taken place via letter or pro forma, and these are still the most appropriate media for non-urgent referrals as copies can be provided for the medical records (both in primary and secondary care). Email communication is replacing the printed word but serves the same purposes. Telephone referral, usually to hospital doctors in the training grades, is appropriate for emergency referral but the process should still be documented. Telephone discussion about a patient can be used as an alternative to referral but it must be clear which clinician retains clinical responsibility,[6] and it would be wise for both parties to document the call and what was said. In a rural setting such as Queensland (Australia), GPs rely on a network of trusted consultants to whom they can turn for both referral and advice, the telephone being the preferred medium.[7] In the UK relationships between GPs and consultants are good, with mutual respect, cooperation and the desire to avoid conflict reported in a qualitative interview study of clinicians in the southwest.[8] There are practical difficulties of course in contacting other clinicians since both GPs and consultants have commitments that preclude immediate availability by telephone.

Telephone contact initiated by consultants to report on the progress or outcomes of patient care was found to be valuable but rare in a literature review conducted by a cardiology department in Pennsylvania (USA).[9] Informing GPs by telephone when children were admitted with acute exacerbations of asthma in Melbourne (Australia), together with a structured discharge summary and follow-up plan, led to greater GP satisfaction with hospital communication.[10]

Telephone consultations between GPs and nurses

Both practice- and community-based nurses need to contact GPs with whom they share the care of patients. Some of this contact takes place face-to-face at the surgery in primary care team meetings and in informal 'corridor' conversations. Practice nurses engaged in treatment room work, minor illness or chronic disease management may need to ask for advice from a medical colleague who is consulting elsewhere in the building, and a community nurse visiting elderly or disabled people at home may need to reach the practice-based doctor. The telephone provides the means of communication in these scenarios. The following transcript represents a real consultation that took place on a Sunday afternoon between a female duty doctor and female hospital nurse attending a patient in the community as part of an early-discharge scheme. The reader is referred to Table 2.3 for an explanation of the transcription notation:

1. hello Missus Collins' residence,
2. oh hello it's Doctor Dawkins here.
3. oh hello=
4. =you rang.
5. hi er my name's (   ) I'm one of the respiratory nurses from the hospital um one of the COPD nurses.
6. right,
7. erm we've got a lady out on our scheme Missus Jane Collins.
8. yeah,
9. she was discharged from hospital nine days ago following an exacerbation of her emphysema.
10. mm mm?
11. erm the day before yesterday she started to feel a bit more [unwell]
12.   [mm mm]
13. resting oxygen sats were (dropped) below ninety per cent
14. [[mm mm]
15. [[(   )] the GP prescribed a dose of clarithromycin two hundred and fifty milligrams [bd
16.   [mm mm]
17.   she] wasn't feeling too bad yesterday but (   ) her resting oxygen saturations are down (0.5) er (   ) we have got an oxygen concentrator here which
18. [[mm]
19. [[we're] using at the moment (0.5) she's got a low grade pyrexia of about thirty seven three continually she's expectorating purulent green sputum=
20. =mm=
21. =and the thing I'm pretty concerned about is her actual spirometry's reduced (0.5) we're doing (   ) spirometry? FEV one's dropped from about fifty four fifty five to about thirty seven=
22. =mm mm=

23. =FVC's dropped from a hundred and thirty to a hundred and sixteen and her peak flow's dropped about er say from about [( )]

[mm]=

24. =seventy er=

25. =is she on nebulisers and things?

26. ( )

27. yeah and she takes some sort of steroid does she?

28. yeah she's on thirty milligrams of pred at the moment.

29. mm right is she actually under hospital care or under GP care then at the moment.

30. what we do is we come out and visit for five days she has erm this er ability ( ) five day and then she=

31. =right=

32. =er so really I mean although I'm still coming out to assess her=

33. =yeah=

34. =she is under the hospital still in some sort of way but obviously it's nurse care and its not just um=

35. =right=

36. =and we're not trained to listen to the chest.

37. [right]

38. [( )] obviously I'm concerned about her (0.5) I have just spoken to my respire well one of the respiratory registrars on call=

39. =yeah=

40. and she said the problem being they've got an acute um problem with beds at the moment up at the hospital=

41. =right=

42. =and it just gone like she's on quite a smallish dose of ( ) probably just just maybe starting amoxicillin as well.

43. right ok what I'll do is ask someone to come and visit then I think,

44. I think=

45. =Dale Drive yeah?=

46. =I think I'd be a lot happier with that.

47. ok then someone will be along.

48. ok do you know roughly how long that will be,

49. ah I think (things are) quieting down a bit now so I don't think it will be terribly long.

50. ok.

51. probably within the hour.

52. ok

53. alright?

54. alright.

55. bye bye.

56. bye bye.

There are several characteristics of inter-professional communication in this example that are worth highlighting, as follows.

Role clarification

In lines 5, 7 and 9 the nurse explains her role, and tries to clarify it later (lines 29–35) while the doctor tries to establish what duty of care she owes to the patient.

Use of jargon

There is a lot of technical language (lines 13–23) and a rather formal manner, implying psychological distance – possibly generated by previous experience or current anticipation of conflict with doctors.

Team-working

The reference to a previous telephone consultation between the nurse and a hospital doctor seems to invoke a decision by the doctor to arrange a home visit, either for an independent assessment or to carry out the recommendations of the hospital-based colleague.

Telephone consultations between GPs and paramedics

Paramedics have skills in assessing and initiating treatment for trauma and acutely ill patients. Although usually based in ambulance services, some paramedics have joined primary healthcare teams and out-of-hours services, extending their role to triage, managing minor illness and giving advice. GPs may meet paramedics face-to-face at the scene of a medical emergency and ambulance crews may contact GPs by telephone from such a scene if they need to hand over a patient. In this example an ambulance crew has assessed a young woman who took an overdose. Medical back-up is requested through the local GP cooperative and a female doctor calls back to speak to the attending male paramedic:

1. **hello?**
2. oh hello it's Doctor Bell=
3. **=[[yeah]**
4.   [[here] hello ringing back about Bethany Docherty?
5. **yeah here.**
6. erm are you the ambulance crew or a friend or a boyfriend?
7. **well the ambulance crew's 'ere.**
8. right well could I speak to them yeah?
9. **yeah.**
10. **hello?**
11. oh hello it's Doctor Bell calling back hello

12. we're just um we're just having a chat with the boyfriend

13. ((doctor: breathy laugh))

14. before we ((chuckling)) go=

15. =right.

16. um yeah the lady with well if you like the family have phoned up via London=

17. =oh God=

18. =the family from London have phoned up er reference an overdose of I think it's hang on carmazzipin erm=

19. =how what's the spelling on that?

20. C-A-R (0.5) B-A-M (0.5) A-Z-E-P (0.5) I-N-E

21. carbamazepine right lovely,

22. yeah.

23. and what strength of the tablets there.

24. have you got the tablets? ((background noise))

25. that's ok.

26. the lady's not actually epileptic er=

27. =[[right   ]

28.   [[boyfriend's] tablets she took the lot and I can't ((background noise)) can you see what dose that is? sorry it's not very good lighting ((patient: ep ep)) it says ep at the end ((patient: a hundred milligrams)) a hundred milligrams.

29. a hundred milligrams

30. we're unsure how many she's taken we know we know for sure she's taken four ibuprofen but apparently she took these last night and there was a hundred and fifty in the bottle=

31. =((doctor tuts))=

32. =but they were prescribed in February and the boyfriend was taking them up till a couple of weeks ago but not at the stated dose so it's all very confusing to get a figure to start with.

33. right.

34. so she's not taken them like in the last few hours (0.5) the residents have gone around the bed and apparently she's been sleeping most of the day she she's not I wouldn't say she's had a conversation with us she's told us where to go and has flatly refused any treatment or anything from us.

35. right ok=

36. =(   )=

37. =what to do and how does she look to you now is she alert and lucid? or is she still sleepy.

38. she's a little bit drowsy but you know she's er she's quite alert to to to any advance we make.

39. is she up and about and moving around?

40. **she's still laying in bed erm she's got a quilt on her but she's quite aggressive to us when we sort of go in the room er we're not really getting a lot of joy you know we thought=**

41. =yeah=

42. **about coming up to the hospital for a check-up but she's not happy to do=**

43. =no=

44. **=one of her friends has just arrived to offer a bit more moral support here but not really (   ) there was a little bit of a domestic disagreement last night which was the trigger.**

45. yeah

46. **that's pretty much all we know about the lady**

47. right ok well from a medical point of view she's likely to be ok now if it's the best part of twenty four hours since the overdose and she hasn't had any problems by now then at this stage the blood levels are gonna be going down quite rapidly so=

48. **=((grunt))=**

49. =I don't think she has to go into hospital=

50. **=right=**

51. =if she's refusing.

52. **right.**

53. I should think the main risk has already passed now anyway I mean if I'd seen her you know last night I almost certainly we would have been pressuring her to go up but um at this point there's probably isn't a lot of point now.

54. **((grunt))**

55. but obviously she needs to be followed up because I mean overdosing's not a sensible thing so we'll probably have to arrange with her own GP to sort of pick that up and try and follow up what needs to be done

56. **by the sound of it there's a little bit of banging and bumping there I would think she's up and out of bed now=**

57. =right=

58. **=shouting**

59. right so there can't be too much wrong with her if she's able to do that

60. **ok**

61. ok so look you=

62. **=what I'll do**

63. right

64. **yeah (   ) I'll advise the boyfriend to contact the surgery in the morning**

65. yeah I would do that we'll fax through a message but if she doesn't want to go I I think at the moment we couldn't really force her because I don't think the risk is high now anyway so you know it's up to her really

66. **(   ) obviously if there's any sort of dramatic changes or any=**

67. =of course=

68. =(   )=

69. =absolutely and likewise here you know if there's any change and they're worried just tell them to give us a call

70. ok

71. it might be easier to call us first if they're worried because then we can assess her and decide without wasting your time.

72. that would be lovely=

73. =yeah [yeah

74.   [thanks very much.

75. um do you want to give them our direct number just in case there is a problem?

76. yeah I've got=

77. two four two four six four? Yeah you've got that?

78. I'll do that.

79. yeah ok.

80. lovely.

81. alright then.

82. thanks.

83. no problem.

84. bye.

85. bye.

This consultation illustrates some additional characteristics of inter-professional dialogue, as follows.

Use of humour

This paradoxical behaviour (lines 13 and 14) is occasionally exhibited between health professionals in the context of trauma and suffering, and is probably a defence mechanism to the stressful situation at hand.

Dealing with relatives

The threat or prospect of having to deal with anxious relatives is expressed by the doctor in line 17. Both this and the earlier laughter help to create social presence.

Joint decision-making

From line 47 the two clinicians work collaboratively, sharing their uncertainty and developing a plan that involves further communication in the short and medium term, depending on the progress of the patient.

Inter-professional communication between out-of-hours services and practices

Information about out-of-hours presentations needs to be communicated to practices in an effective and timely way, especially regarding patients who have been asked to make follow-up arrangements. The National Quality Requirements for out-of-hours service providers stipulate that such information should reach practices by 8:00 a.m. the following working day. Practices need to manage their appointment systems to include capacity for consultations arising from the activities of the out-of-hours service the previous night. One of the conclusions of a study by Marsh *et al.* was the importance of having appointments available at the practice the following morning, which enabled the management of 59 per cent of out-of-hours contacts by telephone alone in Stockton-on-Tees (UK).[11]

Effective communication from practices to out-of-hours service providers prepares colleagues for problems that might arise in patients whose conditions are unstable. Examples include a cancer patient who is terminally ill or a patient with bipolar disorder relapsing into a hypomanic state. Consistency in clinical management between these two aspects of primary care helps to avoid the raising of unrealistic patient expectations. The support of the decisions of a colleague on one shift by a clinician on another demonstrates integration and cooperation between day and night staff. The consultation below took place on a Monday evening between an experienced male GP and a 48-year-old woman. The message taken by the call handler informed the doctor that the patient had consulted her own GP earlier in the day with sinusitis. After presenting her main symptom the patient explains to the second doctor that she had been given a prescription for a broad-spectrum antibiotic:

1. **hello.**
2. oh hello Mister Missus Cohen?
3. **yes yes.**
4. oh hello Doctor Harris here how can I help,
5. **oh it's er I've had er diarrhoea for about four o'clock to seven o'clock continuous and now it's left off a bit but I was put on co-amoxiclav today?**
6. oo:::h dear.
7. **I've only took one tablet the last would that do that?**
8. yes.
9. **and I've had tummy pains like sharp pains (   )=**
10. =what before the co-amoxiclav or after the=
11. **=no after.**
12. oh.
13. **and I've had I don't know it's just like fluid=**
14. =right=

15. =coming away from me=

16. =well it could be the co-amoxiclav or it could be that something else happened to be developing but co-amoxiclav is quite well known for causing diarrhoea how are the sinuses at the moment.

17. **well I'll tell you what I've done I've damaged my cornea and I'm on that lubricating ointment every night?**

18. yeah.

19. **I've had pains in the back of my eyes=**

20. =sure=

21. **=this weekend and I went and she said there was a slight slight swelling down the side of my eyes down=**

22. =right=

23. **=my nose and she thought there was infection=**

24. =oh [right ok]

25.   **[(   )] wanted to give me those=**

26. =oh right well if there's nothing desperately for which you need antibiotics I would stop them and ask your doctor tomorrow.

27. **tomorrow yeah.**

28. yeah.

29. **yeah but would one tablet would that do it? I couldn't imagine that one=**

30. =ooh yes yeah yeah yeah.

31. **it would.**

32. yeah.

33. **and it'd be so fast.**

34. it's unlikely er it's unusual but it's possible yeah.

35. **yeah.**

36. yeah.

37. **you know and I felt violently=**

38. =sure=

39. **=sick and I couldn't be sick.**

40. yeah yeah yeah so so stop the co-amoxiclav,

41. **yeah and just try=**

42. =and see how things are tomorrow yeah.

43. **yeah ok.**

44. ok then.

45. **yeah.**

46. bye.

47. **bye.**

Integration between the patient's daytime and out-of-hours primary care providers breaks down when a doctor criticises his colleague's prescription (lines 6 and 16) and suggests that a medication is not necessary (line 26). The GP does however provide interim advice for the woman's symptoms and encourages her to make further contact with her usual doctor (lines 26 and 42). Advising a patient to stop a drug that appears to be causing significant side effects should not undermine a colleague's efforts if the reasons are explained adequately.

Practical application

Functions of inter-professional telephone consultations and the ways in which inter-professional cooperation and inter-agency integration can be facilitated by telephone are summarised in Box 8.1. Practitioners should be aware of the working hours, routines and availabilities of colleagues in various disciplines in both the primary care team and other agencies in order to find the optimum time to make telephone contact. The task of tracking down a hospital consultant or community psychiatric nurse can be reasonably delegated to a practice receptionist or secretary provided the clinician stands by for the connection to be made.

Box 8.1 Guidance on inter-professional telephone consultations

Functions of inter-professional telephone communication

- To hand over the clinical responsibility for a patient.
- To ask for advice from a colleague with more experience or expertise.
- To refer a patient to secondary care.
- To refer a patient within primary care.
- To share information about a patient.
- To give feedback on an outcome to a colleague.
- To make a shared decision about the management of a patient.
- To organise a specific treatment or procedure.

Inter-professional aspects of telephone consultations with patients

- Be aware of the role and training of primary care team members.
- Support a colleague's reasonable management as far as possible.
- Minimise inconsistency through the use of formularies and protocols.
- Inform patients that part or all of their medical record is to be made available to colleagues involved in their care.
- Exercise additional care to document diagnoses and treatment plans that other health professionals can access and understand.

Exercises

Readers are now invited to consider the roles and duties of professional colleagues through two scenarios, the first where confidential information is sought from a caller and the second where information is given to a team member as part of a referral.

Exercise 15

Objectives: to reflect on aspects of consent and confidentiality in the area of child protection and to enhance team-working skills.

You are a practice nurse and have just finished your morning clinical session when a telephone call is put through to you from a social worker. She is concerned about the safety of a four-year-old boy registered with the practice and is in the process of gathering information for an initial case conference. The child attended recently with an upper respiratory tract infection. His young mother seemed depressed and you encouraged her to make an appointment for herself. The social worker wants to know about the mother's competence as a parent and whether there are any other adults who have contact with the child.

• What are your initial concerns about discussing the boy with the social worker?
• What aspects of inter-professional practice in the area of child protection guide your response to the enquiry?
• How can you work with the primary healthcare team in this situation?

Exercise 16

Objectives: to be able to make a referral to a community nurse taking into account his or her requirements for information and likely approach to the patient's circumstances, and to consider other colleagues who could usefully become involved.

You are a GP on an early afternoon home visit to a frail 86-year-old widow who has called about abdominal pain. She tells you that she has been falling recently and after examining her you conclude that she has a urinary tract infection and constipation with impacted faeces in the rectum. You have given her a prescription for an antibiotic but think that an assessment by your community nurse colleague might also be beneficial to her care. Plan a telephone call to the nurse and consider the following:

• what does the nurse need to know about the patient and her home circumstances?
• what medical information should you convey?
• how will you word your request for help?
• how can the wider primary care team help support this woman through her illness?

References

1. Richards A, Carley J, Jenkins-Clarke S and Richards D. Skill mix between nurses and doctors working in primary care – delegation or allocation: a review of the literature. *International Journal of Nursing Studies* 2000;**37**:185–97.
2. McCallin A. Interdisciplinary practice – a matter of teamwork: an integrated literature review. *Journal of Clinical Nursing* 2001;**10**:419–28.
3. Wilcock P, Campion-Smith C and Head M. The Dorset Seedcorn Project: interprofessional learning and continuous quality improvement in primary care. *British Journal of General Practice* 2002;**52(suppl)**:S39–44.
4. Beck J, Dries T and Cook C. Development of an interdisciplinary, telephone-based care program. *American Journal of Health-System Pharmacy* 1998;**55**:453–7.
5. Saunders J. Handling unexpected distress on the telephone: the development of interdisciplinary training. *International Journal of Palliative Nursing* 2004;**10**:454–9.
6. Cartmill M and White B. Telephone advice for neurosurgical referrals. Who assumes duty of care? *British Journal of Neurosurgery* 2001;**15**:453–5.
7. Hollins J, Veitch C and Hays R. Interpractitioner communication: telephone consultations between rural general practitioners and specialists. *Australian Journal of Rural Health* 2000;**8**:227–31.
8. Marshall M. How well do general practitioners and hospital consultants work together? A qualitative study of cooperation and conflict within the medical profession. *British Journal of General Practice* 998;**48**:1379–82.
9. Haldis T and Blankenship J. Telephone reporting in the consultant–generalist relationship. *Journal of Evaluation in Clinical Practice* 2002;**8**:31–5.
10. Marks M, Hynson J and Karabatsos G. Asthma: communication between hospital and general practitioners. *Journal of Paediatrics & Child Health* 1999;**35**:251–4.
11. Marsh GN, Horne RA and Channing DM. A study of telephone advice in managing out-of-hours calls. *Journal of the Royal College of General Practitioners* 1987;**37**:301–4.

PART 3

Clinical management by telephone

CHAPTER 9

The management of common conditions presenting by telephone

The preceding parts of this book have covered the *process* of telephone consultations conducted by a variety of clinicians and their support staff working in daytime general practice and out-of-hours services. This chapter is about *content* and focuses on fifteen common problems that can be dealt with, at least initially, by telephone:

1. acute febrile illness in children
2. cough and/or breathlessness
3. earache
4. sore and/or discharging eyes
5. rashes and other skin problems
6. spinal pain and injuries
7. other musculoskeletal pain and injuries
8. headache and head injury
9. dental problems
10. diarrhoea
11. cystitis in women
12. vulval and vaginal thrush
13. emergency contraception
14. vaginal bleeding in early pregnancy
15. anxiety and depression.

The limitations outlined in Chapters 2 and 3 should be borne in mind when consulting by telephone: this low-bandwidth communication medium is associated with errors in information transfer for which face-to-face interaction usually compensate; and the decisions made by clinicians are often premature and influenced by time, workload, emotional response and an over-optimistic interpretation of symptoms. Characteristics of the patient are important variables in clinical management, informing clinical judgement as much in telephone consultations as they do in the face-to-face encounter. These variables are:

- age
- gender
- English-language skills
- communication skills
- personal resources
- coping strategies
- pre-existing state of health
- learning disability
- physical disability
- ideas, concerns and expectations
- health beliefs
- culture
- ethnicity
- previous experience of practice/service
- previous consulting behaviour.

Logistical factors also have a profound effect on decision-making, therefore part of any telephone history should include the practical considerations in Table 9.1.

Table 9.1: Logistical factors influencing management in telephone consultations

Patient factors	Availability of a carer
	Care of dependants if patient is a carer
	Transport and capacity to use it
	Confidentiality (e.g. patient calling from work)
Practice factors	Appointment system (capacity, flexibility, skill mix)
	Timetabling (e.g. dedicated telephone consulting session)
	Time of day of call
	Distance between patient and practice
	Contractual considerations
Out-of-hours service factors	Time of day/night (number of professionals available)
	Distance between patient and primary care centre
Locality factors	Dispensing arrangements
	Distance between patient and nearest hospital
	State of traffic (in urban areas)

Each of the 15 common conditions outlined in the sections below will consist of introductory comments and any relevant evidence from the literature followed by the information needed from a caller, factors influencing the triage decision and issues that might arise in negotiation and follow-up. Some conditions benefit from drug treatment either available from a pharmacy over the counter (OTC) or on prescription. OTC medicines that provide symptom relief are appropriate for many acute self-limiting illnesses. For infections that have mixed evidence for the effectiveness of antibiotics, the prescriber should consider the option of issuing a 'delayed' prescription that can be redeemed by the patient at a future date should symptoms not improve spontaneously. Whether prescriptions should be issued on the basis of a telephone history alone is a personal matter for individual practitioners and a policy issue for practices and out-of-hours service providers. Some general principles that should be considered in telephone prescribing are:

- the prescriber should be reasonably confident with the diagnosis reached by telephone
- the patient should be happy to be treated without being seen
- the regular medications taken by the patient and any drug sensitivities should be known or elicited by the clinician
- the treatment should be explained together with its risks and benefits
- adequate provision for follow-up in the event of no improvement, worsening symptoms or side effects should be made
- the patient or a carer should be in a position to attend a pharmacy to obtain the prescribed item
- the drug prescribed should be efficacious, cost-effective and a small quantity issued before reviewing its effects
- controlled drugs should not be prescribed on the basis of a telephone consultation alone.

Acute febrile illness in children

Calls from parents and carers about sick children usually have an element of anxiety,[1] which may or may not be expressed, and this anxiety is often transferred to the health professional receiving the call.[2] In a survey of 146 parents presenting out-of-hours, 49 per cent were driven by a perception of lack of control and 79 per cent expected an explanation or diagnosis to help them make sense of their experience.[3] 'Meningitis' is a common parental concern and meningococcal disease, associated with a potentially fatal form of meningitis, is a condition that GPs fear missing.[4] In interviews doctors described using intuition rather than systematic reasoning under these circumstances and had difficulty complying with guidance to administer parenteral penicillin to patients suspected of having meningococcal sepsis. For babies up to the age of six months, the Baby Check system predicts significant illness[5] but it has had mixed reception in community use.[6,7] Baby Check is a checklist of symptoms and signs each of which is assigned a score. Examples of high-ranking symptoms are a high-pitched or abnormal cry and a fluid intake in the preceding 24 hours of less than one-third of normal. High-ranking signs include bile-stained vomiting and cold hands and feet.

Information needed

How was the temperature assessed or measured?

Some parents judge a child's temperature by touch (forehead, torso), while others use one of a variety of thermometers. Mercury-in-glass thermometers are the most reliable but may be superseded by infrared tympanic thermometers whose sensitivity has been shown to be low in a primary care-based study.[8] High (> 38.5°C) or prolonged (> three days) fevers and those that do not respond to antipyretics may indicate more significant pathology.

What are the associated symptoms?

In the early stages of a febrile illness there may be none, which leads to a high level of diagnostic uncertainty. Respiratory tract infections usually cause one or more of the following cluster of symptoms: sore throat, swollen cervical lymph nodes, runny and/or blocked nose, cough (with or without wheeze) and earache. If the chest seems to be involved then a change in the rate of breathing and any indication that breathing is difficult for the child (e.g. recession in infants) should be asked about. Gastrointestinal infections will manifest as vomiting, diarrhoea or both, but vomiting alone can be a non-specific feature of any illness and should be interpreted with caution. Urinary symptoms may not be present in urinary tract infections in infants and young children, and this diagnosis should be considered in an ill child when fever is the only symptom. Rashes should be asked about together with a description from the caller. Clinicians may obtain clear descriptions of vesicles (suggesting chickenpox) or urticaria (associated with some viral infections), but generalised red macular lesions cannot always be attributed to self-limiting illness. Haemorrhagic skin lesions, a feature of meningococcal septicaemia, can be distinguished from inflamed or hyperaemic ones by the latter's blanching quality: a glass tumbler pressed against the skin will make non-haemorrhagic spots disappear.

What is the general condition of the child?

Information about skin colour, state of alertness and activity, and level of hydration (judged from parental estimation of fluid intake and urine output) help to complete the acute clinical picture. The clinician should ask how far is this a departure from the child's usual state of health. Infants who were born prematurely or children with chronic disease or immune deficiency will be more vulnerable to the effects of infections.

How is the caller feeling/coping/thinking about the problem?

The opportunity for expressing ideas, concerns and expectations should be given to all patients and carers, not just those calling on behalf of children, but the patient- or parent-centred aspects of the telephone history can prove to be valuable in subsequent decision-making. Parents draw upon their experience of previous illnesses, both in the child in question and in its siblings, to judge the potential seriousness of symptoms. Parents' assessments might also be coloured by the prevailing illnesses in the neighbourhood, whether communicable or not.

Triage decision

A face-to-face consultation will be necessary if the child has significant constitutional symptoms, a rash other than a well-described viral exanthem, or if parental anxiety and clinician uncertainty cannot be adequately contained. More important in the triage decision is the conviction in the parent's mind that the ill child needs face-to-face attention. Health professionals conducting telephone consultations should take note of such instincts and, if associated with reasonable concerns, then attendance at the surgery or primary care centre should be offered. Unless there are insurmountable transport or social problems, sick children can be safely taken to the clinician's location.

Telephone management is possible if the condition is likely to be self-limiting and if clinician and caller are prepared to discuss the risks and limitations of a telephone assessment. Whenever possible a diagnosis should be offered together with an explanation of the natural history of the condition. High temperatures in the under-fives are associated with febrile convulsions. The likelihood of this can be reduced by the use of paracetamol or ibuprofen suspension and/or by physically cooling the child with water (tepid sponging or a lukewarm bath). Advice on such supportive treatment and symptom relief should be given together with a description of worsening symptoms that would require further contact. These include pallor, floppiness, reduced urine output, a rising or sustained high fever despite adequate doses of antipyretic medication and the development of a rash.

Negotiation and follow-up

A common issue that might require negotiation is that of antibiotic prescribing.

Antibiotic treatment in uncomplicated upper respiratory tract infection is not indicated.[9] Acute illness in children rarely requires follow-up but there may be situations where arranging a later consultation is appropriate: reassessing a coughing child who may have asthma; supporting a family with psychosocial problems; and administering a vaccination that may be overdue. Other members of the primary care team can be involved with these follow-up scenarios. Before allowing the caller to hang up, he or she should be asked if there are any outstanding questions or concerns.

Cough and/or breathlessness

Coughing often accompanies viral upper respiratory tract infections (URTI) and in the majority of patients is a benign complication that can be managed at home. Coughs in the absence of URTI symptoms need careful assessment because of the lengthy differential diagnosis, which includes:

- inhaled foreign body or irritant
- laryngitis (croup in young children)
- bronchitis (bronchiolitis in babies)
- pneumonia
- asthma/chronic obstructive pulmonary disease (COPD)

- pneumothorax
- malignancy
- pulmonary embolus
- cardiac failure
- side effect of ACE inhibitors.

Breathing problems and coughs can generate non-speech sounds and speech-related signs such as hoarseness, stridor, wheeze or the inability to complete a sentence without drawing breath that can be detected over the telephone. Breathlessness alone may be caused by lung or heart disease, but systemic conditions such as anaemia, thyrotoxicosis and diabetic ketoacidosis should be considered together with psychological problems that might manifest in hyperventilation.

Information needed

Is this a new or recurring problem?

Patients with asthma or COPD may consult during an exacerbation, which may be triggered by a viral infection in the former group or be associated with a bacterial infection in the latter.

Is the cough dry or productive?

Purulent sputum implies bacterial infection (or secondary bacterial infection during a viral illness), blood-stained sputum could be caused by malignancy or pulmonary embolus and white, frothy sputum is associated with pulmonary oedema.

How is the patient's breathing affected?

If wheeze is affecting breathing and the patient is known to be prone to bronchospasm then both the breathlessness and cough should respond to bronchodilator therapy and, if appropriate, oral corticosteroids.

Is there any chest pain?

Lobar pneumonia, pulmonary embolus and pneumothorax frequently cause pleuritic chest pain. Pain on coughing may represent a chest wall muscle tear.

How ill is the patient?

Constitutional symptoms of fever, malaise and confusion, and functional impairments such as the inability to sit or stand, should make the clinician think of sepsis, hypoxia, dehydration or hypotension.

What are the caller's concerns?

Chest symptoms that follow URTIs often lead patients to consult because of anxiety about bronchitis and pneumonia. Physical examination and appropriate reassurance may help coughing patients cope with their symptoms in the knowledge that their chest is 'clear'; others may find it sufficient just to voice their concerns.

Triage decision

A face-to-face consultation is necessary for patients with anything other than URTI with cough, uncomplicated acute bronchitis, acute laryngitis and croup, unless the latter two are associated with stridor. There is evidence that cortico-steroids improve symptoms in children with croup in a hospital environment.[10]

Telephone management is possible for patients with chronic lung disease who have been provided with a peak flow meter and a self-management plan. Some asthma protocols provide for the telephone sanctioning of oral steroid use, while others require that the patient be examined first. Adverse behavioural and psychosocial factors such as alcohol dependency or social isolation should be taken into account before leaving the asthmatic patient to his or her own devices as these are associated with higher mortality.[11] Self-limiting lower respiratory tract infections can be managed with rest, additional fluid intake and steam inhalation. Other breathless patients need a face-to-face consultation for a safe assessment.

Negotiation and follow-up

There may be a patient expectation of an antibiotic prescription or at least a discussion of the possible merits of antibiotics for their condition. The self-limiting causes of cough suitable for management by telephone advice alone do not require antibiotic treatment.[12] Persistent or worsening cough, particularly if breathing becomes affected, should lead to a face-to-face reassessment. Patients calling about exacerbations of asthma and COPD should be invited for a follow-up appointment in order to review their management plans.

Earache

Pain in the ear can be distressing both to patients and carers. Parents naturally wish to help relieve the suffering of their children but it can be difficult to calm a distressed child with earache, particularly in the night. Ear pain as an isolated symptom may be caused by external- or middle-ear disease or referred from a variety of head and neck structures because of the contributions of cranial nerves V, IX, X and cervical root C2 to ear sensation.

Information needed

Is the earache arising in the context of URTI?

Unilateral or bilateral ear pain accompanying or following the onset of URTI can be due to negative middle-ear pressure from Eustachian tube blockage, referred pain from the inflamed naso- or oropharynx or acute otitis media (AOM). Symptoms commonly associated with AOM include discharge, if the tympanic membrane ruptures, and hearing loss. Less commonly AOM is associated with vomiting or loss of balance.

If not, are there any associated ear symptoms?

Itch and/or discharge from the ear in the absence of URTI may be due to acute otitis externa, especially if there is a history of recent swimming, attempting to remove wax or scratching the ear canal.

Has the patient had any previous ear surgery?

Patients with tympanostomy tubes (grommets, T-tubes) may not experience much in the way of pain with ear infections but are more likely to develop a discharge. Pain in an ear that has recently been operated on may represent a complication and requires specialist advice. Problems arising in an only-hearing ear should be taken seriously because of the threat (real or perceived) of complete hearing impairment.

Are there problems with any other head and neck structures?

Conditions as diverse as cervical spondylosis, unerupted wisdom teeth and pharyngeal cancer could potentially present with ear pain.

Triage decision

A face-to-face consultation is advisable for patients with discharging ears and necessary for those with worrying additional symptoms such as vertigo, dysphagia, hoarseness or facial weakness. Children with a long history of ear infections and those with grommets, T-tubes or previous middle-ear surgery should be offered an appointment if the parent or carer requests one. They may be acting on instructions from an ear, nose and throat (ENT) consultant or because of their confidence in the effectiveness of antibiotic therapy.

Telephone management is suitable for those patients with URTI who are in reasonable general condition, even if they have a fever. This is because examination of the ear is unlikely to affect the subsequent management. Pain relief is the most useful treatment in the short term: either paracetamol or ibuprofen for children; paracetamol and codeine for adults.

Negotiation and follow-up

There is marginal benefit in prescribing antibiotics for children with AOM but this is balanced by the risks of allergic reaction and gastrointestinal side effects.[13] The evidence on which this Cochrane review was based has been called into question[14] so the treatment of otitis media remains controversial.

Follow-up is not usually necessary for uncomplicated AOM. Even if the tympanic membrane has perforated, it heals within two weeks in the majority of cases and patients need only be advised to keep the ear dry for this period. AOM may be followed by several weeks of hearing loss due to a persistent middle-ear effusion, but further assessment is not warranted unless the problem persists for three months.

Sore and/or discharging eyes

Patients with conjunctivitis commonly present by telephone, often out-of-hours. The eye is painful or causes irritation, the sclera red or bloodshot and there may be watering or a discharge. It is difficult to distinguish between viral and bacterial infection, and even the former may involve a purulent discharge. Parents calling about children with red or sticky eyes may be concerned about whether play-group or school attendance is permissible, and whether antibiotic treatment is appropriate.

Information needed

Is there an associated viral URTI?

If so, it is likely that eye inflammation is also viral, especially if it is bilateral. Infants may develop unilateral or bilateral eye discharge with URTI if the naso-lacrimal ducts have not yet matured: usually there is no significant conjunctival inflammation and the discharge stops when the cold gets better.

Has the eye been subjected to trauma?

Corneal abrasion is a common injury associated with a persistent foreign-body sensation, watering and photophobia. The defect in the corneal epithelium can be seen with the help of fluorescein and a blue light.

Is there a possibility of a foreign body in the eye?

Special equipment may be needed to remove embedded foreign bodies. Loose parti-cles in the upper conjunctival sac can be seen by everting the upper eyelid and removed by wiping the offending object away with a wisp of clean cotton wool.

Has there been any deterioration in visual acuity?

This will help to distinguish between uncomplicated conjunctivitis and other acute eye conditions that warrant a face-to-face assessment, possibly with an ophthalmologist.

Has there been any recent eye surgery?

Specialist referral or advice may be needed for post-operative complications such as infection or acute glaucoma.

Does the patient wear contact lenses?

They should be removed until the eye complaint has resolved.

Is this a recurring problem, e.g. seasonal?

Allergic conjunctivitis may present in spring and summer in those allergic to pollens, or in response to contact with certain cosmetics.

Triage decision

A face-to-face consultation will be necessary if the patient has a foreign body or if the visual acuity is impaired. Depending on the skills and equipment available at the practice or out-of-hours centre, the consultation may take place either in primary care or at a hospital eye clinic.

Acute infective conjunctivitis may be diagnosed and managed over the telephone in patients with a sore, inflamed, 'gritty' eye or eyes if the history is short and vision uncompromised. The evidence suggests that topical antibiotics are helpful in acute bacterial conjunctivitis.[15] Chloramphenicol eye ointment is now available as an OTC medicine. 'Sticky eye' in infants with URTI should be treated with cool boiled water applied with cotton wool to clean the eyelids and lashes.

Patients calling about probable allergic conjunctivitis may also be directed to a pharmacist in the first instance and offered a later face-to-face consultation if OTC medication fails to control the symptoms.

Negotiation and follow-up

Patients can be invited to contact the practitioner again if symptoms fail to resolve or if visual acuity becomes affected.

Rashes and other skin problems

Allergic responses are common, especially drug reactions. Scabies should be considered when itch, worse at night, is a dominant feature, but this diagnosis is best brought up sensitively in a face-to-face consultation since the condition is associated with significant stigma. There are a few other treatable superficial infections that can be diagnosed by telephone by their characteristic features: impetigo (golden crusts over superficial red lesions), herpes zoster (pain and redness in a dermatome with vesicles) and boils.

Impetigo usually responds to topical fusidic acid or mupirocin but the evidence does not support the routine use of oral antibiotics such as erythromycin and flucloxacillin.[16] Nursery and primary schools often have policies about impetigo, as they do with conjunctivitis, because of its potential to spread between children.

Herpes zoster (shingles) usually affects adults. Systemic antiviral drugs are effective in preventing post-herpetic neuralgia[17] but the evidence is not strong for their efficacy in the acute stage.[18] Shingles affecting the upper division of the trigeminal nerve, and specifically the nasociliary branch, may cause inflammation of the eye and corneal ulceration, in which case ophthalmological advice should be sought.

Boils don't always need to be lanced; some resolve spontaneously by rupturing or regressing while others respond to systemic anti-staphylococcal antibiotics. In parts of the body where the skin is inelastic or has little potential for expansion, even small abscesses may present primarily with pain, for example acute parony-chia and ear canal furuncle.

Bites, stings and other minor wounds may be reported by telephone and a common concern is the risk of tetanus. Patients who have received a total of five doses of tetanus vaccine since birth need no further routine protection. The reader is referred to the Department of Health's 'Green Book'[19] for current guidance on the management of the tetanus-prone wound.

Information needed

What does the lesion or rash look like?
Some diagnoses can be made from a clear description.

Is the lesion single or are there multiple lesions?
If multiple then the distribution of the rash may reveal a recognisable pattern.

What are the associated symptoms, if any?
Local symptoms such as pain, itch and discharge should be asked about as well as constitutional symptoms that might indicate systemic disease of which the rash is a manifestation.

To what has the patient been exposed?
A drug history may help if no obvious environmental trigger emerges from the history.

If the lesion is a boil at what stage is it?
A boil with a yellow or white head can be encouraged to rupture by applying heat, for example with a clean cloth soaked in hand-hot water; one that has already ruptured may be managed with absorbent dressings.

Triage decision

Any very ill person with a rash should be examined because meningococcal septicaemia is always a possibility. Telephone management is possible if a diagnosis can be made and the community pharmacist available for those requiring antihistamine treatment, a soothing cream or a supply of dressings.

Negotiation and follow-up

Adverse drug reactions should be recorded and the clinician should consider reporting the side effect to the Committee on Safety of Medicines (www.mca.gov.uk/ [accessed November 2006]). Follow-up should be offered to all patients with skin lesions that fail to resolve with home remedies.

Spinal pain and injuries

Pain arising from the spine and its associated structures is a common presentation in primary care. Adults of working age, irrespective of occupation, are vulnerable to both acute and chronic spinal pain, and the causes are usually benign; investigation and/or emergency admission are rarely necessary.

Most calls about acute neck and back pain will be for advice on or practical help with pain control, and/or sick leave from work. There is little difference in the effectiveness of the various modalities of treatment aimed at relieving low-back[20] or neck pain[21] and episodes are usually self-limiting.

Information needed

How mobile is the patient?

Stiffness, deformity and inability to move the head in neck pain or walk in low-back pain are associated with more severe injuries, usually to soft tissues but potentially to facet joints and intervertebral discs. The muscle spasm associated with some spinal injuries contributes to the pain experienced by the patient.

Are there any 'red flags'?[22]

Older patients (> 55) with new neck or back pain, as opposed to an acute exacerbation of chronic pain, and young patients (< 20) with spine pain should be assessed more carefully since the differential diagnosis includes malignancy in both age groups and developmental abnormalities in the latter. The pain may radiate in the distribution of a nerve root but numbness or parasthesia in a dermatome may represent significant nerve root compression. Questions aimed at excluding spinal cord or cauda equina compression should be asked: 'Is there bilateral lower limb weakness and/or numbness?' and 'Is there loss of or impaired sphincter function?'

Is the patient capable of work?

Back pain is a common cause of absence from work.

What analgesia has the patient tried so far and what is available in the home?

Non-steroidal anti-inflammatory drugs (NSAIDs) are first-line treatment and some patients respond to paracetamol combined with a mild opioid drug such as codeine.

Triage decision

A face-to-face consultation will be necessary if there are red-flag symptoms or if more potent analgesia is likely to be needed. The mobility of the patient will dictate whether the consultation takes place at the surgery/primary care centre or at the patient's home. Telephone management is possible if the history is short, even if the patient is unfit for work. It can be difficult to predict the natural course of the condition in any individual so certification can be left until the seventh day of absence. It is legitimate to issue a medical certificate to a patient after a telephone consultation, but a prolonged episode of spinal pain should be managed with face-to-face contact.

Negotiation and follow-up

Plain radiography has been shown to be unreliable in acute spinal pain but patients often request an X-ray. GPs still refer patients[23] despite the evidence.[24] It should be possible to explain that such images, which require a significant dose of radiation, rarely influence the management of uncomplicated neck or low-back pain while remaining supportive of the patients and addressing his or her concerns. Persistent or worsening spinal pain despite analgesia justifies a face-to-face assessment and consideration of a referral to a physiotherapist or to a specialist with access to CT or MRI scanning facilities.

Other musculoskeletal pain and injuries

Patients with limb injuries should be assessed by telephone for their severity, functional impairment and risk of complications in order to distinguish between those patients that require accident and emergency (A&E) department attendance or community nurse assessment from those that patients and carers can manage themselves. Practices that provide a minor injuries service as part of their GMS contract[25] may invite patients to be assessed and treated at the surgery. Falls are a common cause of trauma in the elderly, and management should include a falls risk assessment and the correction of predisposing environmental and pathological factors.

Information needed

Was the onset of the pain or impairment spontaneous?

Spontaneous joint pain occurs in patients with a metabolic or rheumatic predisposition such as gout and arthritis. There may be a history of overuse, prolonged weight bearing or unusual movement in the affected limb or limbs and the joint may be described as hot, swollen, stiff or a combination of these. Septic arthritis is associated with malaise and fever, and is a medical emergency. Pain in a prosthetic joint may be difficult to assess but if it occurs in the first few weeks after surgery infection should be considered.

Spontaneous pain and swelling in the lower limb raises the possibility of deep venous thrombosis (DVT). Predisposing factors include prolonged immobility, previous or family history of DVT, and combined oral contraceptive use.

Was the onset of the pain or impairment the result of an injury?

The mechanism of the injury will give the clinician an indication of the likely structures that absorbed the force of the trauma.

Does the patient need the services of an A&E department?

Direct referral to A&E may be made for suspected fractures (bony tenderness, swelling, deformity and loss of function) and other injuries that require specialist assessment such as function-threatening hand trauma, burns and multiple injuries.

Has the patient been deliberately injured and are they safe?

Dependent elderly, disabled adults and all children may be injured deliberately by their carers, so the history of trauma arising in a social context should include a tactful enquiry about the possibility of abuse. In some cases, particularly children, such questions may put the victim at greater risk. GPs should be familiar with the procedures in their locality for the protection of children and not hesitate to express their concerns to a duty social worker.

Is the patient able to look after himself or herself and is there a suitable carer?

Elderly or frail patients dependent on carers may develop greater needs than can be managed in the home as a result of an injury. They may need to be admitted to hospital or have their care package reviewed.

Triage decision

A face-to-face consultation will be necessary in patients with suspected infection, DVT, fracture or whose injuries are caused by abuse or assault. For patients who are unable to attend the surgery or primary care centre, the options include a home visit or direct referral to hospital. Adult victims of assault may not need a face-to-face consultation for the treatment of their injuries *per se* but the clinician may be required at a later date to generate a statement for the police based on observations made when the patient presented.

Most musculoskeletal problems can be managed by telephone advice. Pain relief advice includes non-pharmacological strategies such as the application of an ice pack and elevation of the affected limb. Management other than analgesia depends on the disability caused by the condition. Elderly patients living alone may need temporarily to recruit a relative or neighbour to help with their activities of daily living and personal safety. Those without such resources may need referral to community nurses or social services.

Negotiation and follow-up

There may need to be some discussion about the logistics of providing additional care to dependent patients, depending on the resources available at the time of the telephone consultation. Hospital admission for nursing care may allow time for extra home care arrangements to be made.

Headache and head injury

The differential diagnosis of spontaneous headache includes tension headache, migraine, temporal arteritis, subarachnoid haemorrhage, meningitis and malignant hypertension. A common technique used by doctors to help them discriminate between the head pain caused by subarachnoid haemorrhage from other headaches is to ask, 'Is this the worst headache you have ever had?' Although a positive response to this question should lead to emergency admission for CT scanning and lumbar puncture, its specificity is around 10 per cent,[26] the more common cause of a sudden severe headache being benign 'thunderclap' headache.[27]

Classic migraine headaches are unilateral, often centred over or around the eye, severe in intensity, throbbing in nature and associated with nausea and vomiting, and in some cases visual disturbances (zigzag lines, photophobia). Patients often have a family history and certain foods or stress may trigger an attack.

There is a growing incidence and concern about medication-overuse headache,[28] therefore the history in an acute presentation should include a review of painkiller use before perpetuating the problem by advising more medication. Strategies such as rest, relaxation and herbal remedies may encourage patients to seek non-pharmacological therapies for subsequent headaches. The 'doctor as drug' concept described by Balint[29] is applicable to the management of headache: it has been shown that one of the factors predicting the resolution of headache is the opportunity that the patient has to discuss his or her problem fully with the family doctor[30] or a specialist.[31]

Information needed

What are the characteristics of the headache?

Descriptions of the distribution of the pain, its nature, severity and how these change throughout the day are required, together with any response to home remedies. The patient's speech may reveal a confusional state or more specific neurological signs such as dysarthria or dysphasia.

Is this a new or recurring problem?

Migraine sufferers occasionally call with particularly severe attacks, especially when their usual strategies have failed to relieve symptoms or when their psychosocial circumstances lower their threshold for seeking help. For a first attack in a woman, it is important to establish whether she is using the combined oral contraceptive pill, since focal migraine is a contraindication to its use.

For spontaneous headache, what are the associated symptoms?

Neck stiffness and photophobia are the cardinal signs of meningeal inflammation or irritation and the possibilities of meningitis and subarachnoid haemorrhage should be considered. Raised intracranial pressure may cause nausea and vomiting. Acute febrile illnesses may be associated with headache.

For head injuries, what are the associated symptoms?

A period of unconsciousness or amnesia, pallor, drowsiness and vomiting may represent brain injury.

What concerns does the patient have?

Headaches have a variety of meanings for patients, for example stress, high blood pressure, meningitis and brain tumour.

Triage decision

Physical examination is required for patients whose conscious level is impaired, those with meningitis-like symptoms, migraine sufferers with prolonged pain and vomiting, and anyone with suspected raised intracranial pressure.

Telephone management is possible for patients with minor head injuries, defined as those with a Glasgow Coma Scale[32] score of 15, but this must include informing the patient or carer about the worsening symptoms of drowsiness, vomiting and confusion that might suggest raised intracranial pressure. For a comprehensive guideline, including the telephone assessment of head-injured patients, the reader is referred to the National Institute for Clinical Excellence.[33]

Negotiation and follow-up

Hypertension is common but rarely causes headache. A presentation of headache may include a discussion about blood pressure and the opportunity should be taken at some stage to measure the blood pressure if this has not been done in the past year.

Dental problems

Emergency dental presentations are:[34]

- severe acute continuous pain
- recent onset or increasing swelling of the gum
- bleeding, e.g. from the site of a recent extraction
- trauma, e.g. tooth knocked out
- malaise following dental treatment.

Information needed

Is the patient registered with a dentist or had dental treatment recently?

Some patients may not have contacted their dentist or the local emergency dental service, while others may have tried but not been able to arrange an appointment. Provision of out-of-hours dental care for unregistered patients was found to be lacking in over two-thirds of health authorities in the UK in a survey published in 2000.[35] Calls from patients with acute dental problems were subjected to a triage protocol in a trial based in a North Wales GP cooperative and found to be effective and satisfactory to patients.[36] The protocol provided practitioners with the means to direct callers to a dental support line and give names of local dentists for them to consult.

How does the pain respond to simple analgesics?

Severe pain may reflect the presence of pus or an exposed nerve.

Are there any worrying features?

These would include fever, trismus, dysphagia and airway obstruction.

Triage decision

A face-to-face consultation will be necessary for patients who are bleeding, have dental or jaw problems as a result of an injury, or who have any of the worrying features outlined above. If an emergency dental service for unregistered patients is available in the locality then this would be the most appropriate setting for the consultation. In the absence of such a service primary care clinicians may find it helpful to consult their hospital-based maxillofacial surgery colleagues by telephone for advice or referral.

Usually the only therapeutic option available to the GP or practice nurse is to prescribe antibiotics and NSAIDs. Whether this happens with or without a face-to-face appointment will be a matter for clinical judgement. Amoxicillin is the antibiotic of choice, metronidazole being a second-line option for the penicillin-allergic patient.

Negotiation and follow-up

If antibiotic therapy is initiated it is important that the patient consult with a dentist at the earliest opportunity rather than relying on the prescription as a substitute for definitive care.

Diarrhoea

Diarrhoea is the frequent passage of unformed stools. This symptom can occur in all age groups and can be accompanied by vomiting. When diarrhoea and vomiting coincide, the risk of dehydration increases. Those most vulnerable to dehydration are the very young and very old. Common causes are viral gastroenteritis and food poisoning.

Information needed

Is this a rapid-onset gastrointestinal disturbance with a likely environmental cause?

A short history of diarrhoea following exposure to another person with similar symptoms or to contaminated food is likely to be consistent with a diagnosis of infective diarrhoea, a self-limiting but extremely unpleasant illness caused by both viruses (e.g. rotavirus in children) and bacteria (e.g. campylobacter). A caller may have acquired an infection abroad, increasing the range of possible pathogens to include amoeba and *Giardia*.

What is the patient's state of hydration?

The balance between fluid intake and fluid loss is difficult to assess over the telephone, especially with babies and young children still in nappies because urine output can be impossible to assess when all the diapers contain liquid stool. An older child or adult who has passed little or no urine in the last twelve to 24 hours may be dehydrated. Postural dizziness may be also reported in the history. Parents and carers of young children may notice loss of skin turgor or sunken eyes. While the anterior fontanelle remains palpable, it can be used as a guide to the circulating volume, the sagittal venous sinuses being just deep to it. A sunken fontanelle is a sign of significant hypovolaemia, of which dehydration is one cause.

How vulnerable is this patient to the effects of dehydration?

Pre-existing health problems or frailty influence the patient's capacity to compensate for fluid loss. Patients who depend on regular medication may not be able to absorb the drugs properly when they have diarrhoea. This is particularly important in patients on long-term corticosteroids, the sudden withdrawal of which may increase sodium and water loss.

Is there any associated abdominal pain?

Colicky pain may be present but constant or severe pain warrants a physical examination, since diarrhoea can be a presenting symptom for appendicitis, colitis and infective exacerbations of diverticular disease.

Triage decision

A face-to-face consultation will be necessary if the patient is, or is likely to become, significantly dehydrated, or is suspected to have an acute abdomen that requires hospital admission.

Telephone treatment should be limited to those otherwise fit patients who have diarrhoea, or diarrhoea plus vomiting, with or without colicky abdominal pain. Instructions should be given about rehydration using glucose and electrolyte solutions available from the pharmacist. Antidiarrhoeal drugs such as loperamide can also be purchased OTC but should not be used by children. Probiotic treatment may be worth advising.[37]

Negotiation and follow-up

Gastroenteritis and infective diarrhoea are usually self-limiting infections and prescriptions are rarely necessary. Patients with prolonged symptoms and those with diarrhoea acquired abroad or from food should have a sample of their stool analysed by the local Health Protection Agency laboratory. Antibiotics may benefit returning travellers[38] and metronidazole could be prescribed without waiting for the result of a stool culture. Antibiotics are not effective in patients with *Salmonella*.[39] Patients who work with food will be required to stay away until their symptoms have resolved and may therefore require a medical certificate.

Cystitis in women

There is evidence to support the treatment of uncomplicated urinary tract infection (UTI) in women by telephone.[40,41] The first of these studies from the USA evaluated an algorithm for the management of dysuria or urgency in the absence of nausea, fever and vaginal discharge. Women were treated with an antibiotic (trimethoprim, nitrofurantoin or ciprofloxacin) according to symptoms without laboratory investigation. In the second, 72 patients were randomised to receive either telephone or office-based management. All participants had their urine cultured and two-thirds of the results were positive. All in the telephone group and all but two patients in the control group were treated with antibiotics. Avoiding a face-to-face consultation is convenient for women but limits diagnostic accuracy.[42]

Information needed

Is the patient pregnant or could she be?

UTI in pregnancy is more likely to affect the upper urinary tract and may precipitate premature labour. Some antibiotics often used for UTI are contraindicated (trimethoprim) or not advised in pregnancy (quinolones).

Do the symptoms refer to acute inflammation of the bladder?

It is important to establish in a telephone history whether a woman's discomfort is coming from her bladder rather than her vulva or vagina. It can be difficult to distinguish between cystitis, sexually transmitted urethritis and *Candida* infection. Antibiotic treatment aimed at curing a UTI may not be sufficient to treat an STI (sexually transmitted infection) and may make thrush worse.

Are there any associated symptoms?

Fever is unusual in uncomplicated UTI and should lead the clinician towards a diagnosis of acute pyelonephritis, especially if the woman is also experiencing rigors, vomiting or loin pain. The presence of blood in the urine reflects the degree of inflammation but need not influence management.

What treatment has the patient tried so far?

Most women are aware that cystitis can be treated symptomatically with home remedies or alkaline salts from the pharmacy.

Triage decision

Patients may have had previous experience of UTI and usually make their own diagnosis. If a woman is presenting with her first UTI then it is appropriate to ask her to provide a mid-stream urine specimen for laboratory microscopy and culture, but this needn't involve a face-to-face consultation. Empirical antibiotic treatment can be started once the specimen has been provided.

Negotiation and follow-up

If alkaline drinks have not yet been tried then it is reasonable to advise these. If this plan is not acceptable to the patient or it has been unsuccessful then it is safe to offer antibiotic therapy provided there is no history of adverse reaction to the intended drug. A prompt response to antibiotics should be expected so failure to respond within 24–48 hours would be a reason for review. If a laboratory test has been organised then the patient will need to know how the result will be made available or conveyed to her.

Vulval and vaginal thrush

This can arise spontaneously, as a result of increased frequency of sexual intercourse or a change of sexual partner, or as a side effect of broad-spectrum antibiotic treatment. It is more common in pregnancy.

Information needed

Is the patient pregnant or could she be?

Thrush is harmless to the fetus. However, the fetus might be harmed by prescribed drugs.

Are the symptoms predominantly vulval (soreness, itch, superficial dyspareunia) or vaginal (pain, thick white or cream-coloured discharge, deep dyspareunia) or both?

This will help determine the most appropriate treatment.

Are there any constitutional symptoms?

Occasionally diabetes will present with thrush owing to the condition's effect on immunity.

Has the symptom arisen from intercourse with a new partner?

If thrush is transmitted sexually then other STIs may be present but asymptomatic or masked by the thrush.

What has the patient tried so far?

Some women may have used topical antifungal preparations (cream and/or pessary); others may find OTC treatment prohibitively expensive.

Triage decision

A face-to-face consultation is advisable for patients with recurrent thrush, or symptoms suggestive of thrush that have failed to resolve with appropriate OTC medication. These women may need an examination and laboratory test of a swab to help with the diagnosis.

Telephone management is safe if the diagnosis is clear from the history, and the patient is otherwise well. If the patient has not tried topical antifungals, then these can be obtained from a pharmacist or prescribed. Oral fluconazole is an alternative and has been shown to be equally as effective.[43]

Negotiation and follow-up

A single dose of fluconazole taken by mouth is more acceptable to women than the use of creams and pessaries[43] but more expensive, therefore the practitioner may need to balance patient preference and convenience against managing resources. Most patients only require follow-up if their symptoms do not resolve or recur soon after treatment.

Emergency contraception

Women who have had unprotected sex often consult about emergency contraception by telephone instead of in person. The consultation should include a discussion about the risks of having acquired an STI.

Information needed

Is the patient pregnant or could she be?
The date of the last period will help to determine this.

Have there been any other episodes of unprotected sex in the current cycle?
Treatment will only be effective for unprotected intercourse in the preceding five days.

How long ago was the most recent episode?
Women presenting within 72 hours may be eligible for emergency oral contraception. Those making contact between three and five days after intercourse may need to be considered for a post-coital coil insertion.

What are the woman's usual contraceptive arrangements and are they satisfactory to her?
This may lead to a decision to review contraception at a later stage.

Triage decision

A face-to-face consultation will be necessary if the patient considers herself at risk of STI or if she is not eligible for oral therapy. It is appropriate to offer women the choice of being treated by the practice or out-of-hours service, attending a family-planning clinic or purchasing post-coital contraceptive tablets from a pharmacist, who will also provide appropriate counselling.

The treatment involves two doses of 0.75mg of levonorgestrel 12 hours apart within 72 hours of intercourse. Patients unlikely to remember the second dose can be advised to take both doses at once.[44] This can be prescribed without seeing the patient. A study in North Carolina (USA) to increase access to emergency contraception found that a strategy of telephone consultations and faxed prescriptions to pharmacists succeeded in providing treatment to over 7000 patients in a two-and-a half-year period.[45]

Negotiation and follow-up

Occasionally a clinician will speak to a patient who has been treated with levonorgestrel several times, which may reflect a need for more reliable contraception. Care should be taken to assess the patient's perspective and insight as it is important to remain non-judgemental.

Emergency contraception is no guarantee against unplanned pregnancy. Women for whom post-coital contraceptives are prescribed should report back if their next period does not start within a week of its expected date.

Vaginal bleeding in early pregnancy

The threat of a miscarriage in the early stages of a wanted pregnancy through the development of bleeding in the first trimester is distressing to women and their partners. Ultrasound scanning has become the standard form of assessment of viability of the fetus.[46] The administration of anti-D to Rhesus negative women is no longer thought necessary for bleeding in the first trimester.[47] Scanning should also help to identify those women with ectopic pregnancy but if this condition is suspected from the history a direct referral to a gynaecologist is preferable.

Information needed

When was the patient's last menstrual period and has a pregnancy test been positive?
Hospital ultrasound departments and duty gynaecologists will require this information.

How heavy is the bleeding?
Although difficult to estimate, the patient should be able to compare the blood loss with her normal periods. Very heavy bleeding may require emergency treatment and hence a face-to-face assessment.

What is the nature of any associated pain?
Cramping period-like pain may indicate that the contents of the uterus are being expelled and constant unilateral pelvic pain should alert the clinician to the possibility of a rupturing tubal pregnancy.

Have products of conception been passed?
The patient may describe a sac or the fetus itself, which would suggest that the miscarriage is complete, especially if the bleeding and any associated pain are beginning to subside.

How is the woman feeling emotionally?
Some patients seem to cope with the threat of miscarriage, while others are intensely distressed. Her partner, if present, may also be anxious.

Triage decision

Patients may be referred for ultrasound without the need to meet face-to-face, provided the woman is otherwise well and can either take herself or be reliably transported to hospital. A face-to-face consultation will be necessary if the health of the patient is at risk from haemorrhage that threatens her circulation or from infection, with a view to making a referral to the on-call gynaecologist. Speculum inspection of the cervix can help in the diagnosis of bleeding in early pregnancy but physical examination can potentially precipitate rupture of a tubal pregnancy, hence the reluctance of many GPs to examine women with a suspected ectopic pregnancy.

Negotiation and follow-up

It can be difficult for the patient to accept advice to rest and wait for the outcome of an ultrasound scan in the case of a threatened miscarriage. Distress and anxiety may be managed better by a home visit or attendance at the surgery/primary care centre. If the patient has already 'booked' her pregnancy, the midwife should be informed of the problem in order not to make her next contact expecting all to be well. If the pregnancy is viable then antenatal care can continue as normal.

Anxiety and depression

Acute psychological problems and exacerbations of pre-existing psychiatric morbidity, including personality disorders and substance misuse, may lead to telephone consultation between affected patients or carers and their primary care team or an out-of-hours service. The suitability for managing a patient's crisis by telephone will depend on how well the patient and his or her psychosocial circumstances are known.

Information needed

Is this an acute or longstanding problem?

If acute, it is helpful to find out what has precipitated the current crisis.

Is the patient's mental state reasonable under the circumstances?

Practitioners need to be careful not to medicalise the 'normal' stresses and moods experienced in life but to remain alert for cues that indicate the patient is not coping.

Is the patient intoxicated?

This will make mental-state examination difficult and may limit management options. A history of substance or alcohol misuse may either be a cause or an effect of anxiety and depression.

Is the patient at risk of harming themselves or others?

Suicide risk should be signposted and assessed with straightforward questions. It is common for patients in distress or with depression to have fleeting suicidal thoughts but persistent invasive ideas, fantasies or even specific plans of suicide are pathological and an indication for psychiatric intervention. The social context of the presentation should be established in order to identify other people, particularly children, at risk of harm.

What sources of support are already available?

Family and friends may be willing to support the patient through a crisis or an acute exacerbation of a mental illness. If the patient is on psychotropic medication there may be scope for a temporary increase in the dose, for example to aid sleep. Other professionals in both primary and secondary care may be involved with the case and there may be an accessible key worker who knows the patient well.

Triage decision

Telephone management should be restricted to those patients without suicidal ideas, adequate social support and whose distress is understandable given the context. These patients may improve without a prescription, the opportunity to share their feelings having considerable therapeutic benefit. The telephone can be used to perform an initial mental-state examination since the tone, pace and content of his or her speech can be detected adequately this way. The patient's posture, any abnormal movements, appearance, clothing, personal hygiene and willingness to make eye contact can only be assessed face-to-face.

Self-help materials and information are available for patients on a variety of mental-health issues from Mind (www.mind.org.uk/Information/Factsheets/ [accessed November 2006) and increasingly via interactive websites.

Negotiation and follow-up

Agitated and suicidal patients may be best assessed at their current location rather than a GP surgery or out-of-hours primary care centre since there is a risk that other patients may be disturbed. If the visiting practitioner is at risk of assault or if it is likely that the patient will need to be admitted compulsorily, then the local police may need to be informed and possibly involved.

Under less dramatic circumstances, patients can be given tasks to perform before their follow-up appointment, such as writing down more about their symptoms, weighing up the pros and cons of a particular behaviour, considering which relationships are helping and which are harming their mental state, or even completing a validated instrument such as Goldberg's General Health Questionnaire.[48]

Practical application

The 15 presentations described above have been summarised into single-page boxes for quick reference to readers. It is difficult to provide guidance that can be universally applied because patients do not usually fall into neat categories, and patient and logistical factors will affect one's clinical judgement. Readers will be able to use the guidance to ensure they cover the main issues and to provide safe advice. When the guidance advises face-to-face consultation this could take place in either primary or secondary care, in the latter case by direct referral or by advising the patient to attend the nearest A&E department.

Although the guidance has been reduced to a checklist of bullet points, it is not intended that the clinician use them as a basis for the structure of their telephone interviews. Rather, in the process of gathering information through the appropriate use of open and closed questions, he or she includes the key points at naturally occurring opportunities within a patient-centred dialogue that addresses both biomedical symptoms and the illness experience.

Box 9.1 Guidance on the telephone management of acute febrile illness in children

Information needed
- What is the temperature?
  - method of measurement
  - reliability of method
  - duration of temperature
  - changes over time.
- What are the associated symptoms?
  - none
  - respiratory/gastrointestinal/urinary
  - rash.
- What is the general condition of the child?
  - colour/activity/warm or cold extremities
  - feeding and drinking/urine output
  - changes over time.
- What are the parent's/carer's ideas and concerns?
  - fear of grave diagnosis
  - unanswered questions.

Telephone management appropriate if
- diagnosis fairly clear
- infection is self-limiting
- child in reasonable condition
- no rash apart from viral exanthema
- caller willing to accept reassurance and advice.

Telephone advice
- Increase fluid intake.
- Antipyretic medication.
- Physical cooling measures.
- Worsening symptoms requiring further contact:
  - child develops signs of dehydration
  - child develops a rash (if no viral exanthema at initial contact)
  - temperature increases further.

Face-to-face consultation appropriate if
- diagnosis uncertain
- infection likely to require intervention
- child in poor condition
- non-specific or unrecognisable rash
- caller unwilling to accept reassurance and advice.

Box 9.2 Guidance on the telephone management of cough and/or breathlessness

Information needed

- Is this a new or recurring problem?
    - preceding URTI
    - pre-existing chronic lung disease.
- Is the cough dry or productive?
    - purulent/blood-stained/frothy.
- How is the patient's breathing affected?
    - respiratory rate
    - wheeze
    - recession.
- Is there any chest pain?
    - constant
    - on inspiration (pleuritic)
    - on coughing.
- How ill is the patient?
    - sepsis/hypoxia/dehydration/hypotension.
- What are the caller's concerns?
    - bronchitis/pneumonia.

Telephone management appropriate if

- acute self-limiting viral URTI or LRTI
- no significant constitutional symptoms
- wheezy breathlessness in a known asthma or COPD patient with a self-management plan.

Telephone advice

- Rest.
- Increase fluid intake.
- Steam inhalation.
- Antipyretic medication, if applicable.
- Worsening symptoms requiring further contact:
    - constitutional symptoms develop
    - respiratory distress/increasing respiratory rate.

Face-to-face consultation appropriate if

- breathlessness without wheeze in an asthma or COPD patient
- risk factors for asthma mortality
- breathlessness is a new symptom
- stridor in croup or laryngitis
- significant constitutional symptoms.

Box 9.3 Guidance on the telephone management of earache

Information needed

- Is the earache arising in the context of URTI?
- If not, are there any associated ear symptoms?
    - discharge/itch
    - hearing loss/vertigo.
- Has the patient had any previous ear surgery?
    - tympanostomy tubes
    - eardrum repair.
- Are there problems with any other head and neck structures?
    - cervical spine (C2)
    - wisdom teeth/sinuses (V)
    - pharynx/larynx (IX, X).

Telephone management appropriate if

- earache arises in context of URTI
- antibiotics are not indicated and caller happy with this, OR
- 'wait and see' approach to antibiotics is acceptable to caller.

Telephone advice

- Analgesia (paracetamol, ibuprofen, codeine).
- Keep ear dry for patients with otitis externa.
- Worsening symptoms requiring further contact:
    - pain persists or intensifies despite analgesia
    - worrying features develop.

Face-to-face consultation appropriate if

- ear is discharging
- ear is vulnerable (only hearing ear, previous surgery)
- worrying features (vertigo, hoarseness, dysphagia, facial weakness)
- antibiotics or hospital referral are indicated.

Box 9.4 Guidance on the telephone management of sore and/or discharging eyes

Information needed

- Is there an associated viral URTI?
- Has the eye been subjected to trauma?
- Is there a possibility of a foreign body in the eye?
    - corneal abrasion is associated with a foreign-body sensation.
- Has there been any deterioration in visual acuity?
- Has there been any recent eye surgery?
- Does the patient wear contact lenses?
- Is this a recurring problem, e.g. seasonal?

Telephone management appropriate if

- history is consistent with acute conjunctivitis:
    - infective/allergic
- the visual acuity has not changed.

Telephone advice

- Bathing an infant's sticky eyes.
- OTC medicines:
    - antiseptic ointment
    - chloramphenicol ointment
    - sodium cromoglycate
    - artificial tears.
- Prescribed medicines:
    - other antibiotic ointment or drops.
- Worsening symptoms requiring further contact:
    - if unilateral, the other eye becomes involved
    - visual acuity deteriorates.

Face-to-face consultation appropriate if

- the diagnosis is uncertain
- trauma was involved or a foreign body may be present
- there is a reduction in visual acuity
- referral to an ophthalmologist is likely.

Box 9.5 Guidance on the telephone management of rashes and other skin problems

Information needed
- What does the lesion or rash look like?
    - vesicular/pustular/macular/urticarial/pigmented.
- Is the lesion single or are there multiple lesions?
    - dermatome/trunk/limbs/flexures.
- What are the associated symptoms, if any?
    - itchy/painful/weeping/crusted/constitutional symptoms.
- To what has the patient been exposed?
    - drugs/chemicals/foods/viruses/plants/insects/animals.
- If the lesion is a boil at what stage is it?
    - pointing/discharging.

Telephone management appropriate if
- sepsis can be reasonably excluded in the history
- a reversible environmental cause can be identified
- OTC treatments or home remedies are acceptable
- the condition is expected to resolve spontaneously.

Telephone advice
- OTC medicines:
    - antihistamine for allergic reactions
    - 10 per cent crotamiton or 1 per cent hydrocortisone cream for itchy lesions
    - dressings.
- Exposure avoidance.
- Worsening symptoms requiring further contact:
    - lesion or rash spreads
    - lesion or rash becomes infected
    - patient becomes unwell.

Face-to-face consultation appropriate if
- diagnosis not clear from caller's description
- the patient is unwell
- surgical intervention may be required, e.g. incision of an abscess
- prescribed drugs may be required, e.g. antivirals, potent topical steroids.

Box 9.6 Guidance on the telephone management of spinal pain and injuries

Information needed
- How mobile is the patient?
    - walking
    - limping/not weight-bearing
    - bed bound.
- Are there any red flags?
    - age > 55/age < 20
    - limb weakness/sphincter disturbance
    - night pain/weight loss.
- Is the patient capable of work?
    - self-certificate/medical certificate/self-employed.
- What analgesia has the patient tried so far and what is available in the home?
    - non-steroidal anti-inflammatory drugs
    - paracetamol and codeine.

Telephone management appropriate if
- the history is short (< 1 week)
- no red flags
- analgesia is accessible and adequate.

Telephone advice
- Mobilise the spine.
- Change position frequently.
- Apply heat or icepacks.
- Regular analgesia.
- Worsening symptoms requiring further contact:
    - pain more severe or unresponsive to drugs
    - limb weakness or numbness
    - urinary retention or incontinence.

Face-to-face consultation appropriate if
- the history is long (> 1 week)
- one or more red-flag features are present
- home remedies or OTC analgesics are insufficient
- referral to a physiotherapist or consultant may be required.

Box 9.7 Guidance on the telephone management of other musculoskeletal pain and injuries

Information needed

- Was the onset of the pain or impairment spontaneous?
    - arthritis prosthetic joint
    - risk factors for DVT.
- Was the onset of the pain or impairment the result of an injury?
    - mechanism of injury.
- Does the patient need the services of an A&E department?
    - fracture/dislocation
    - neurovascular trauma/risk of permanent impairment.
- Has the patient been deliberately injured and are they safe?
    - abuse/assault/ongoing risk.
- Is the patient able to look after himself or herself and is there a suitable carer?
    - social history and functional assessment.

Telephone management appropriate if

- mechanism of injury unlikely to cause fracture/dislocation/permanent impairment.

Telephone advice

- Rest initially, then mobilise.
- Apply ice pack.
- Elevate if swollen.
- Analgesia.
- Worsening symptoms requiring further contact:
    - increasing pain/swelling
    - further loss of movement/function
    - signs of infection
    - signs of impaired circulation.

Face-to-face consultation appropriate if

- treatment is provided in primary care for minor injuries
- hospital assessment or admission is likely.

Box 9.8 Guidance on the telephone management of headache and head injury

Information needed

- What are the characteristics of the headache?
    - unilateral/band-like/occipital/bitemporal
    - throbbing/constant/worse in mornings.
- Is this a new or recurring problem?
    - analgesic use/history of migraine.
- For spontaneous headache, what are the associated symptoms?
    - nausea/vomiting
    - neck stiffness/photophobia.
- For head injuries, what are the associated symptoms?
    - amnesia/vomiting/drowsiness.
- What concerns does the patient have?
    - intracranial haemorrhage/brain tumour/hypertension.

Telephone management appropriate if

- the history suggests:
    - tension headache
    - migraine
    - minor head injury.

Telephone advice

- Rest.
- Relaxation.
- Analgesia (unless patient is overusing).
- Worsening symptoms requiring further contact:
    - drowsiness
    - vomiting
    - confusion
    - meningism.

Face-to-face consultation appropriate if

- the history suggests:
    - impaired conscious level
    - meningism
    - prolonged migraine attack
    - raised intracranial pressure.

Box 9.9 Guidance on the telephone management of dental problems

Information needed
- Is the patient registered with a dentist or had dental treatment recently?
    - assess access to emergency dental services
    - complications of dental treatment:
        - bleeding/malaise.
- How does the pain respond to simple analgesics?
    - if little response or none consider:
        - infection/exposed nerve.
- Are there any worrying features?
    - fever/trismus/dysphagia/airway obstruction.

Telephone management appropriate if
- no worrying features
- care can be taken over or continued by dentist.

Telephone advice
- Analgesia:
    - NSAIDs/paracetamol and codeine.
- Antibiotic:
    - amoxicillin/metronidazole.
- Advise patient to contact dentist at first available opportunity, OR
- provide patient with information about emergency and routine access to dental care.
- Worsening symptoms requiring further contact:
    - symptoms deteriorate despite treatment
    - worrying features develop
    - patient unable to register with a dentist.

Face-to-face consultation appropriate if
- bleeding or history of trauma
- one or more worrying features present
- referral to hospital oral surgeon likely.

Box 9.10 Guidance on the telephone management of diarrhoea

Information needed
- Is this a rapid-onset gastrointestinal disturbance with a likely environmental cause?
    - exposure to another person with diarrhoea
    - contaminated food source.
- What is the patient's state of hydration?
    - urine output/postural dizziness
    - skin turgor/anterior fontanelle.
- How vulnerable is this patient to the effects of dehydration?
    - extremes of age
    - comorbidity
    - medication, e.g. corticosteroids.
- Is there any associated abdominal pain?
    - constant/colicky
    - mild/moderate/severe.

Telephone management appropriate if
- patient is usually fit and well
- able to tolerate oral fluid
- any abdominal pain is mild or moderate and colicky.

Telephone advice
- Rehydration with glucose and electrolyte solutions.
- Avoid infecting others.
- Antidiarrhoeal drugs:
    - loperamide 4 mg stat then 2 mg after each loose stool.
- Stool specimen for culture for:
    - prolonged symptoms
    - food workers
    - returning travellers.
- Antibiotics:
    - metronidazole in returning travellers 400 mg tds for five days.
- Worsening symptoms requiring further contact:
    - dehydration
    - colicky pain intensifies or becomes constant.

Face-to-face consultation appropriate if
- patient is likely to be, or at risk of becoming, dehydrated
- referral for assessment of the acute abdomen is likely.

Box 9.11 Guidance on the telephone management of cystitis in women

Information needed

- Is the patient pregnant or could she be?
    - increased likelihood of ascending infection
    - limits choice of antibiotic.
- Do the symptoms refer to acute inflammation of the bladder?
    - vaginal discharge/vulval inflammation.
- Are there any associated symptoms?
    - fever/vomiting/loin pain/blood in the urine.
- What treatment has the patient tried so far?
    - analgesia/additional fluids/alkaline salts.

Telephone management appropriate if

- cystitis is uncomplicated.

Telephone advice

- Alkaline salts (potassium citrate) made up into drinks.
- For first episode mid-stream urine specimen for laboratory microscopy and culture.
- Antibiotic treatment:
    - trimethoprim/nitrofurantoin/cefalexin/amoxicillin.
- Advice on prevention, e.g. pass urine after intercourse.
- Worsening symptoms requiring further contact:
    - no response to antibiotic
    - development of fever and/or loin pain.

Face-to-face consultation appropriate if

- UTI precipitates premature labour
- pyelonephritis is likely.

Box 9.12 Guidance on the telephone management of vulval and vaginal thrush

Information needed

- Is the patient pregnant or could she be?
- Are the symptoms predominantly vulval?
    - soreness/itch/superficial dyspareunia.
- Vaginal?
    - pain/thick white or cream-coloured discharge/deep dyspareunia.
- Or both?
- Are there any constitutional symptoms?
    - malaise/thirst/weight loss.
- Has the symptom arisen from intercourse with a new partner?
- What has the patient tried so far?
    - topical antifungal/natural yoghurt.

Telephone management appropriate if

- diagnosis is clear from history
- concurrent STI unlikely
- no constitutional symptoms.

Telephone advice

- Topical antifungal:
    - vaginal – clotrimazole pessaries 500 mg once or 200 mg daily for 3 days
    - vulval – clotrimazole cream 1 per cent apply bd or tds for 3 to 5 days
- OR, oral antifungal:
    - fluconazole 150 mg stat.
- Advise patient to inform sexual partner, who may also require treatment.
- Worsening symptoms requiring further contact:
    - no response to treatment
    - constitutional symptoms develop.

Face-to-face consultation appropriate if

- vaginal swabs are indicated
- recurrent episodes
- risk of concurrent STI
- adequate treatment has failed
- constitutional symptoms are present.

Box 9.13 Guidance on the telephone management of emergency contraception

Information needed

- Is the patient pregnant or could she be?
  - last menstrual period.
- Have there been any other episodes of unprotected sex in the current cycle?
  - more than 72 hours ago
  - more than five days ago.
- How long ago was the most recent episode?
- What are the woman's usual contraceptive arrangements and are they satisfactory to her?

Telephone management appropriate if

- patient eligible for oral treatment.

Telephone advice

- Levonorgestrel 0.75 mg tablets:
  - one tablet stat followed by one 12 hours later, OR
  - two tablets in a single stat dose.
- Spotting may occur after two or three days.
- Next period may be a few days early or late.
- Worsening symptoms requiring further contact:
  - report if next period one week overdue.

Face-to-face consultation appropriate if

- risk of STI
- unprotected intercourse more than 72 hours ago.

Box 9.14 Guidance on the telephone management of vaginal bleeding in early pregnancy

Information needed
- When was the patient's last menstrual period and has a pregnancy test been positive?
- How heavy is the bleeding?
    - spotting/like a period/heavier than a period.
- What is the nature of any associated pain?
    - mild/moderate/severe
    - colicky/constant
    - midline/unilateral.
- Have products of conception been passed?
    - sac/fetus/placental fragments.
- How is the woman feeling emotionally?
    - available support.

Telephone management appropriate if
- patient is otherwise well
- bleeding no heavier than a period
- pain is absent or midline, mild and cramping.

Telephone advice
- Rest.
- Fetal viability ultrasound scan to be arranged.
- Worsening symptoms requiring further contact:
    - pain more severe
    - bleeding heavier
    - pain to one side.

Face-to-face consultation appropriate if
- patient is unwell
- bleeding is heavier than a period
- pain is moderate or severe and cramping
- any lateralised pain.

Box 9.15 Guidance on the telephone management of anxiety and depression

Information needed

- Is this an acute or longstanding problem?
    - past psychiatric history/pre-morbid personality/collateral history
    - drug and alcohol history/prescribed medication.
- Is the patient's mental state reasonable under the circumstances?
    - bereavement/relationship or financial problem/stress at work.
- Is the patient intoxicated?
    - slurred speech/disinhibition.
- Is the patient at risk of harming themselves or others?
    - suicidal ideation or intent/threats to others.
- What sources of support are already available?
    - friends/relatives/key worker.

Telephone management appropriate if

- mental-state examination can be carried out (apart from appearance)
- there is no risk of suicide or self harm
- the patient has insight into the problem.

Telephone advice

- Listening.
- Brief psychological interventions:
    - reframing/homework/leaflets.
- Adjust medication temporarily.
- Worsening symptoms requiring further contact:
    - increasing anxiety
    - deepening depression
    - thoughts of self-harm or suicide develop.

Face-to-face consultation appropriate if

- there is a risk of self-harm or suicide
- the patient is intoxicated (delay appointment until sober)
- new medication is indicated
- referral or admission to hospital is likely to be required.

Exercises

In keeping with the multi-disciplinary approach of this book, there follow exercises that allow primary care teams to plan responses to several common presentations and one rare one.

Exercise 17

Objective: to design care pathways that facilitate multi-disciplinary practice in telephone management for common clinical problems.

Write protocols that could be followed by a nurse or paramedic working in your practice for the telephone management of the following:

- an otherwise fit young adult with:
    - a sore throat
    - a minor head injury
- a sexually active woman:
    - who has forgotten a dose of combined oral contraceptive
    - two weeks late with her period who thinks she may be pregnant
- a parent whose pre-school child has developed:
    - a widespread, itchy, vesicular rash after a sore throat and a cough
    - head lice
- a request from a county council refuse collector for a medical certificate for less than seven days' absence from work with back pain
- a request for a repeat prescription for antidepressants from a head teacher who has been reviewed by her doctor in the previous month.

Exercise 18

Objective: to formulate a response to a media health scare that threatens the running of a practice or out-of-hours service provider.

A teenage boy becomes unwell at school and is admitted to the local hospital's intensive care unit with suspected meningococcal septicaemia. The local evening newspaper carries a report with the headline 'Pupil has meningitis bug: hundreds exposed' and includes the advice that worried parents should contact their GP. Plan a practice or out-of-hours service strategy for managing a series of telephone enquiries from and about people who may or may not have had contact with the affected boy. In particular:

- how would you access information about the nature of the boy's disease?
- who would you ask for expert advice on post-exposure prophylaxis, assuming the diagnosis is meningococcal septicaemia?
- how would you apply the advice to anxious callers?
- how would you manage the practice or out-of-hours team in order to continue providing a service to other callers?

References

1. Kai J. What worries parents when their preschool children are acutely ill, and why: a qualitative study. *British Medical Journal* 1996;**313**:983–6.
2. Foster J, Jessop L and Dale J. Concerns and confidence of general practitioners in providing telephone consultations. *British Journal of General Practice* 1999;**49**:111–13.
3. Kallestrup P and Bro F. Parents' beliefs and expectations when presenting with a febrile child at an out-of-hours general practice clinic. *British Journal of General Practice* 2003;**53**:43–4.
4. Brennan C, Somerset M, Granier S, Fahey T and Heyderman R. Management of diagnostic uncertainty in children with possible meningitis: a qualitative study. *British Journal of General Practice* 2003;**53**:626–31.
5. Morley C, Thornton A, Cole T, Hewson P and Fowler M. Baby Check: a scoring system to grade the severity of acute systemic illness in babies under 6 months old. *Archives of Diseases in Childhood* 1991;**66**:100–6.
6. Kai J. 'Baby Check' in the inner city – use and value to parents. *Family Practice* 1994;**11**:245–50.
7. Thomson H, Ross S, Wilson P, McConnachie A and Watson R. Randomised controlled trial of effect of Baby Check on use of health services in first 6 months of life. *British Medical Journal* 1999;**318**:1740–4.
8. Hay A, Peters T, Wilson A and Fahey T. The use of infrared thermometry for the detection of fever. *British Journal of General Practice* 2004;**54**:448–50.
9. Arroll B and Kenealy T. Antibiotics for the common cold and acute purulent rhinitis (Cochrane Review). *The Cochrane Library, Issue 3*. Chichester, UK: John Wiley & Sons, Ltd, 2004.
10. Russell K, Weibe N, Saenz A, Ausejo Segura M, Johnson D, Hartling L, *et al*. Glucocorticoids for croup (Cochrane Review). *The Cochrane Library, Issue 4*. Chichester, UK: John Wiley & Sons, Ltd, 2004.
11. British Thoracic Society and Scottish Intercollegiate Guidelines Network. *British Guideline on the Management of Asthma: A national clinical guideline*. www.brit-thoracic.org.uk/docs/asthmafull.pdf [accessed November 2006]. April 2004.
12. Smucny J, Fahey T, Becker L and Glazier R. Antibiotics for acute bronchitis (Cochrane Review). *The Cochrane Library, Issue 3*. Chichester, UK: John Wiley & Sons, Ltd, 2004.
13. Glasziou PP, Del Mar CB, Sanders SL and Hayem M. Antibiotics for acute otitis media in children (Cochrane Review). *The Cochrane Library, Issue 3*. Chichester, UK: John Wiley & Sons, Ltd, 2004.
14. Bain J. Treatment of acute otitis media: are children entered into clinical trials representative? *British Journal of General Practice* 2001;**51**:132–3.
15. Sheikh A, Hurwitz B and Cave J. Antibiotics versus placebo for acute bacterial conjunctivitis (Cochrane Review). *The Cochrane Library, Issue 4*. Chichester, UK: John Wiley & Sons, Ltd, 2004.
16. Koning S, Verhagen A, van Suijlekom-Smit L, Morris A, Butler C and van der Wouden J. Interventions for impetigo (Cochrane Review). *The Cochrane Library, Issue 4*. Chichester, UK: John Wiley & Sons, Ltd, 2004.
17. Johnson RW and Dworkin RH. Treatment of herpes zoster and postherpetic neuralgia. *British Medical Journal* 2003;**326**:748–50.
18. Lancaster T, Silagy C and Gray S. Primary care management of acute herpes zoster: systematic review of evidence from randomized controlled trials. *British Journal of General Practice* 1995;**45**:39–45.
19. Department of Health. *Immunisation against Infectious Disease*. London: Department of Health, 1996.
20. Assendelft W, Morton S, Yu E, Suttorp M and Shekelle P. Spinal manipulative therapy for low-back pain (Cochrane Review). *The Cochrane Library, Issue 4*. Chichester, UK: John Wiley & Sons, Ltd, 2004.
21. Gross A, Hoving J, Haines T, Goldsmith C, Kay T, Aker P, *et al*. Manipulation and mobilisation for mechanical neck disorders (Cochrane Review). *The Cochrane Library, Issue 4*. Chichester, UK: John Wiley & Sons, Ltd, 2004.

22. The Guideline Development Group. *Clinical Guidelines for the Management of Acute Low Back Pain*. London: The Royal College of General Practitioners, 2001.
23. Hollingworth W, Todd C, King H, Males T, Dixon A, Karia K, *et al*. Primary care referrals for lumbar spine radiography: diagnostic yield and clinical guidelines. *British Journal of General Practice* 2002;**52**:475–80.
24. Waddell G, McIntosh A, Hutchinson A, Feder G and Lewis M. *Low Back Pain Evidence Review*. London: The Royal College of General Practitioners, 1999.
25. The NHS Confederation. *Investing in General Practice: The new General Medical Services Contract*. London: The NHS Confederation, 2003.
26. Van Gijn J. Subarachnoid haemorrhage: diagnosis, causes and management. *Brain* 2001;**124**:249–78.
27. Giffin N. Sudden headaches. *CPD Journal of Acute Medicine* 2004;**3**:17–21.
28. Diener H and Limmroth V. Medication-overuse headache: a worldwide problem. *Lancet Neurology* 2004;**3**:475–83.
29. Balint M. *The Doctor, His Patient and the Illness*. London: Pitman Medical, 1968.
30. The Headache Study Group of the University of Western Ontario. Predictors of outcome in headache patients presenting to family physicians – a one year prospective study. *Headache* 1986;**26**:285–94.
31. Fitzpatrick R and Hopkins A. Effects of referral to a specialist for headache. *Journal of the Royal Society of Medicine* 1983;**76**:112–15.
32. Teasdale G and Jennett B. Assessment of coma and impaired consciousness: a practical scale. *Lancet* 1974;**2**:81–4.
33. National Institute for Clinical Excellence. Clinical Guideline 4. *Head Injury: Triage, assessment, investigation and early management of head injury in infants, children and adults*. London: NICE, 2003.
34. Jones C. When is toothache an emergency? *The New Generalist* 2003;**1**:23–5.
35. Anderson R and Thomas D. Out-of-hours dental services: a survey of current provision in the United Kingdom. *British Dental Journal* 2000;**188**:269–74.
36. Horton M, Harris R and Ireland R. The development and use of a triage protocol for patients with dental problems contacting an out-of-hours general medical practitioner cooperative. *Primary Dental Care* 2001;**8**:93–7.
37. Allen SJ, Okoko B, Martinez E, Gregorio G and Dans LF. Probiotics for treating infectious diarrhoea (Cochrane Review). *The Cochrane Library, Issue 3*. Chichester, UK: John Wiley & Sons, Ltd, 2004.
38. De Bruyn G, Hahn S and Borwick A. Antibiotic treatment for travellers' diarrhoea (Cochrane Review). *The Cochrane Library, Issue 3*. Chichester, UK: John Wiley & Sons, Ltd, 2004.
39. Sirinavin S and Garner P. Antibiotics for treating salmonella gut infections (Cochrane Review). *The Cochrane Library, Issue 3*. Chichester, UK: John Wiley & Sons, Ltd, 2004.
40. Saint S, Scholes D, Fihn S, Farrell R and Stamm W. The effectiveness of a clinical practical guideline for the management of presumed uncomplicated urinary tract infection in women. *American Journal of Medicine* 1999;**106**:636–41.
41. Barry H, Hickner J, Ebell M and Ettenhofer T. A randomised controlled trial of telephone management of suspected urinary tract infections in women. *Journal of Family Practice* 2001;**50**:589–94.
42. Flach S, Longenecker J, Tape T, Bryan T, Parenti C and Wigton R. The relationship between treatment objectives and practice patterns in the management of urinary tract infections. *Medical Decision Making* 2003;**23**:131–9.
43. Watson M, Grimshaw J, Bond C, Mollison J and Ludbrook A. Oral versus intra-vaginal imidazole and triazole anti-fungal agents for the treatment of uncomplicated vulvovaginal candidiasis (thrush): a systematic review. *British Journal of Obstetrics and Gynaecology* 2002;**109**:85–95.
44. Faculty of Family Planning and Reproductive Health Care Clinical Effectiveness Unit. *FFPRHC Guidance Emergency Contraception*. www.ffprhc.org.uk/admin/uploads/EC%20revised%20PDF%2019.06.03.pdf [accessed November 2006]. 2003.

45. Raymond E, Spruyt A, Bley K, Colm J, Gross S and Robbins L. The North Carolina DIAL EC project: increasing access to emergency contraceptive pills by telephone. *Contraception* 2004;**69**:367–72.
46. Sotiriadis A, Papatheodorou S and Makrydimas G. Threatened miscarriage: evaluation and management. *British Medical Journal* 2004;**329**:152–5.
47. Royal College of Obstetricians and Gynaecologists. *Use of Anti-D Immunoglobulin for Rh Prophylaxis*. London: Royal College of Obstetricians and Gynaecologists, 2002.
48. Goldberg D. *General Health Questionnaire (GHQ 12)*. Windsor, UK: NFER-Nelson, 1992.

CHAPTER 10

Telemedicine

Alternatives to the telephone consultation

The term 'telemedicine' encompasses a variety of medical activities, the common theme being geographical separation of the participants. Contemporary telemedicine makes use of interactive audio, video or other electronic media to deliver health care. The term includes the processes of diagnosis, treatment, transfer of medical data such as images, inter-professional consultation and medical education, for example the teaching of surgical procedures. The European Commission's healthcare telematics programme defines telemedicine as: 'rapid access to shared and remote medical expertise by means of telecommunications and information technologies, no matter where the patient or relevant information is located'.[1] Access to medical expertise can either occur in real time or asynchronously, so-called 'store-and-forward' telemedicine. Patients on the whole are satisfied with real-time interactive video consultations[2] but this qualitative systematic review included only two primary care-based studies in its 32 eligible papers, one of which was cited in Chapter 2 as a clinical example of cuelessness[3] and the other only involved seven patients.[4] An example of store-and forward telemedicine is given by a remote management system designed for the asthmatic children of US military personnel stationed in the Pacific islands.[5] A web-based tool together with video clips to assess inhaler technique led to improved clinical outcomes for a small sample of seven children. This chapter provides the reader with examples of telemedicine applications and summarises broader forms of distant consultation via email, text telephones, interactive telephony and mobile telephones.

Cost-effectiveness

It is difficult to find evidence to support the cost-effectiveness of telemedicine because of the heterogeneity of media, disciplines, healthcare systems and contexts, especially geographical. Whitten and colleagues undertook a systematic review of over 600 articles that included cost in telemedicine.[6] They concluded that there was no evidence to demonstrate the cost–effectiveness of telemedicine initiatives. Through the subsequent correspondence it was acknowledged that intangible costs and benefits exist, including quality of life issues for both patients and clinicians. A US telemedicine programme has been successfully managing diabetic patients for many years through attention to the structures, processes and outcomes of chronic disease management.[7] Telemedicine has advantages for rural primary care.[8] In the UK the Virtual Outreach Project Group conducted a randomised controlled trial of joint teleconsultations involving over 2000 patients in both urban and rural settings. Fewer investigations were ordered in the intervention group and these patients were more satisfied with their experience[9] but the authors calculated that virtual outreach consultations cost £100 more than conventional referrals.[10] Time rather than financial cost was the outcome measure in a study of a telemedicine service for patients with peripheral vascular disease that enabled patient, community nurse and vascular surgeon to consult as a virtual team.[11] The teleconsultations took a mean of 10 minutes compared with the 15 minute face-to-face consultations. The costs of telemedicine systems are likely to fall in the future and therefore the cost–benefit ratio will improve. Readers may wish to explore the potential advantages and disadvantages of the various systems for their own organisations, so suggestions are made in the exercises at the end of the chapter.

Cardiology

Telemedicine needn't just involve health professionals. Eisenberg and colleagues reported on an experiment to increase the proportion of patients with out-of-hospital cardiac arrest receiving bystander basic life support.[12] Callers to emergency services in a suburb of Seattle (USA) were offered on-the-spot training in cardiopulmonary resuscitation (CPR) over the telephone by emergency dispatchers. The study demonstrated a moderate increase in bystander-initiated CPR after the intervention and the authors estimated that four lives had been saved over two years.

Accounts of electronic links between primary and secondary care to help in referral decisions about patients with chest pain or arrhythmias illustrate the benefits of this technology. The transmission of ECGs from 456 patients with suspected life-threatening cardiac events to a hospital-based cardiologist in Italy saved 28 admissions.[13] The sensitivity and specificity of the GPs' clinical diagnosis was 47 per cent and 76 per cent respectively, but it was assumed that the consultant's diagnosis was always correct. The characteristics of the specialist's assessment was calculated in another Italian study that included a teleconsultation as well as the patient's ECG. This telecardiology service performed with a sensitivity of 97.4 per cent and a specificity of 89.5 per cent.[14] Less helpful is the use of telemedicine in the diagnosis of atrial fibrillation: the interpretation of the heart sounds of 60 elderly volunteers heard by six senior family medicine residents with the patients was compared with the interpretation of the same observers listening at a distance through the use of an electronic stethoscope. There was no difference in the diagnostic accuracy of either form of examination.[15]

Dermatology

A group from Manchester (UK) compared teleconsultation with a distant dermatologist followed by a traditional face-to-face consultation in 126 patients referred
by their GPs.[16] As well as demonstrating patient satisfaction the authors estimated
that only 50 per cent of the referrals need have involved a face-to-face consultation
with a specialist and that 75 per cent of the teleconsultations were of educational
benefit to the referring doctors. Where both types of consultation resulted in a single diagnosis there was a highly statistically significant level of agreement.
'Teledermatology' is still in its infancy[17,18] but represents the sort of medicine-at-a-
distance that GPs will become more involved in as the technology develops and
becomes cheaper. Currently patients find the process satisfactory[19] but their GPs
remain unsure.[20]

Gynaecology

Etherington *et al.* designed a service for women with cervical cytology abnormalities in Birmingham (UK) that involved telecolposcopy.[21,22] Practice nurses were
trained to take recordings using a video-colposcope and transmit them to the
gynaecologist. By comparing findings in 81 women by traditional outpatient col-
poscopy with the telemedicine method, sensitivity and specificity were found to be
88.9 per cent and 93.3 per cent respectively.

Psychiatry

Because the mental-state examination can be conducted remotely, telemedicine techniques have been applied to psychiatric and psychological problems. As early as the
1950s Wittson (University of Nebraska, USA) began using two-way closed-circuit
television for the assessment and treatment of psychiatric patients.[23] The administration of diagnostic and screening instruments can be done as reliably by telephone
as in person for research purposes.[24] Telepsychiatry is feasible according to a 2002
literature review[25] but a study from London demonstrated that patients took longer
to complete treatment when managed by videoconferenced psychiatric consultations between a primary care centre and a community mental-health centre.[26]

Telecare

An Audit Commission report on assistive technologies[27] defines telecare as personal
care based around a patient's home in which a variety of functions are controlled
remotely with various technologies and which provide communications to the outside world. Telecare systems allow people to retain their independence through
admission avoidance, virtual visiting, reminder and security systems.[28] NHS Direct is
planning a response to the National Service Framework for Long-Term Conditions.[29]
Chronic-disease management will become an information-based system exploiting
not only telecommunications but also information technology in general for the
benefit of patients (Dr Nicholas Robinson, NHS Direct, personal communication).

Email

In 2002 a sample of patients and GPs in a Leeds (UK) practice were asked whether their face-to-face consultation could have been dealt with by telephone or by email.[30] The doctors thought that more consultations could have been conducted at a distance compared with patients, but in only 3.5 per cent of consultations did both patient and doctor agree that telephone would have been a satisfactory alternative medium and in only 2.2 per cent of consultations was there agreement about email communication. The study had a methodological problem in that patients completed their questionnaire before the consultation and the GP afterwards but is consistent with the findings of an earlier UK study on predicting which GP consultations could be booked as telephone appointments.[31] Ten per cent of patients who used email for other purposes (representing 52 per cent of the sample) communicated with doctors via this medium in a 1999 survey conducted in a Michigan (USA) academic primary care department.[32] The authors expressed concern at their subjects' complacency about security and confidentiality.

The telephone has satisfied the needs of both clinicians and patients in a variety of clinical and administrative encounters for nearly 130 years. Electronic communication has not been adopted as widely in medicine as a consultation medium because of concerns over workload implications[33] and security.[34] Early adopters of email communication with patients argued that such consultations are more easily documented, allow time for a more considered response, can be worded more discreetly and are cost-effective compared to their telephone equivalent.[35] A Scottish practice found that providing a clinical email service did not affect workload and was welcomed by patients.[36] Two-hundred-and-four US physicians who frequently use email to communicate with patients were surveyed about their experiences.[37] Commonly reported email topics were new, non-urgent symptoms, and questions about lab results. Twenty-five per cent of the doctors in this sample were dissatisfied with email as a communication medium for patients. Spielberg, an ethicist from Harvard Medical School (USA), examined the legal and ethical issues of email communication in medicine that affect trust in the doctor–patient relationship: informed consent should be obtained from patients and documented; encryption software should be used to prevent interception of messages and therefore break confidentiality; and email communications should be suitable for inclusion in the medical record.[38]

Web chat is a variation on the email theme that allows real-time communication over the internet, usually within a circumscribed area of cyberspace called a chat room. Some web chat interactions are supplemented by web cam images (digital camera attached to each participant's computer). The Clinical Enquiry Service provided by NHS Direct Online (www.nhsdirect.nhs.uk/index.aspx [accessed November 2006]) was evaluated recently.[39] Twenty-five patients were asked to test the service before seeing their GP about non-urgent problems. The median duration of the web chat sessions was 30 minutes, twice that of NHS Direct telephone calls. There was agreement between remote nurse assessment and GP in 45 per cent of cases.

Text telephones

Email can be used by people with impaired speech or hearing. An alternative technology is the text telephone, which transmits typed messages along telephone lines. The method relies on there being text telephone facilities at both ends of the lines, so practices and out-of-hours providers would need to invest in special equipment in order to provide this service to those patients and carers with special communication needs.

Interactive telephony

It is not uncommon nowadays for practices to manage incoming telephone calls with an automated system that invites the caller to navigate a 'tree' of options depending on the nature of the call. For example:

> Welcome to High Street Surgery. Doctors Brown, White and Green are consulting today together with nurse Pat. If you are calling about a medical emergency please press 1 now. If you wish to make an appointment please press 2. If you wish to arrange a repeat prescription please press 3. If you wish to find out the results of tests please press 4. For all other queries please hold and a receptionist will be with you shortly.

These systems are helpful for large and busy practices that deploy reception and clerical staff in specific tasks for timetabled periods. Time is saved by eliminating the need for a human being to transfer the call to an appropriate colleague. Telephone service providers will install such systems and customise them to suit the practice. Patients may find automatic switchboards impersonal and a barrier to access, but they also meet them in other situations such as when calling hospitals, banks and telecommunications companies. Interactive telephony not only assumes that patients have touch-tone telephones but also that their reasons for contacting their GP fall into neat categories.

More complex programmes allow the caller to enter data or even speech into the computer at the other end of the line. Health applications include the playing of recorded messages about health promotion and disease management, which a patient can choose from a menu, or the collection of information from patients such as a blood glucose reading or mental state.[40] Kobak and colleagues' study compared the use of a screening instrument administered in person, by telephone and by interactive telephony to psychiatric outpatients, with groups of patients from primary care, alcohol treatment centres and eating disorder services, and with healthy controls. Human and computer assessments compared favourably and patients were more honest about their alcohol intake when interacting with the machine. In another US study in primary care depressed patients were more likely to take their antidepressants when an interactive system was introduced.[41]

Mobile telephones

Practices that make outgoing telephone calls to patients and carers will find their telephone bills increasing as a greater proportion of patients are using their mobile telephones as their main or only means of telecommunication. GPs make use of the technology in order to keep in touch with their practices and to triage calls while out on visits.

Mobiles also have a short message service (SMS or text facility). A rheumatologist reported on several examples of the use of text messaging such as informing patients about the results of investigations and allowing patients to report urgent concerns and new or changed symptoms.[42] A multi-disciplinary team led by a GP adopted this communication medium to remind young asthmatics to take their inhalers.[43]

Cellular telephones can now be used to send and receive emails, images and video clips, access the internet, and transmit and facilitate the wireless transfer of data to personal digital assistants and computers. The potential for harnessing these applications to health care is considerable, but they may create greater distance between patients and their professional carers as they conduct their business in an increasingly virtual world.

Practical application

The telephone consultation is just one example of a range of remote contacts between patients and health professionals. Remote consultations take advantage of information and communications technology so that physically distant patients and clinicians – even whole healthcare teams – can participate in information-sharing and joint decision-making. Through electronic and wireless connections data other than speech can be transmitted and the introduction of videoconferencing has added back some of the visual cues lacking in speech-only communication. Telemedicine has a place at the interface between primary and secondary care, and primary care teams need to consider and be prepared to incorporate these alternatives to the traditional referral. Box 10.1 contains a summary of telemedicine applications relevant to primary care.

Exercises

Exercise 19

Consider taking advantage of your patients' mobile telephones by sending results or reminders to them using text messages. To be sure that the practice has the correct number, a brief test message can be sent to ask for confirmation of the patient's identity. Since it is possible for third parties to see the transmitted information, special attention will have to be paid to obtaining informed consent from patients.

Box 10.1 Guidance on the applications of telemedicine in primary care

Advantages

- Costs offset by intangible benefits:
    - reduces time and costs involved in patient travel, e.g. rural areas
    - patient participation and satisfaction generally high
    - educational benefit to referring clinician.
- Suitable for a range of hospital disciplines.
- Store-and-forward methods are time efficient.

Disadvantages

- Probably not cost-effective.
- Set-up costs expensive:
    - videoconferencing equipment in dedicated room.
- Transmission of data potentially insecure.
- Real-time methods are time-consuming.

Telecare

- Suitable for elderly or disabled patients in social isolation.
- Through assistive technologies seeks to:
    - avoid acute admission to hospital
    - enhance personal and home security
    - facilitate chronic disease management.

Email

- Consultations easily documented.
- Responses need not be in real time.
- Cost-effective.
- Potentially insecure.

Text telephones

- For speech- or hearing-impaired patients.
- Requires identical equipment in practice.

Interactive telephony

- Automated switchboard.
- Impersonal but in widespread use in other service sectors.

Mobile telephones

- Text messaging to remind patients about making appointments, taking medication, etc.

This method would only be suitable for people whose mobile telephones are for their personal use and kept with them at all times. Even if the text message is seen only by the intended recipient, it will be stored unless deleted, leaving the patient and practice vulnerable to breaches of confidentiality.

- Undertake a feasibility study by canvassing opinion from your practice manager, reception staff, practice nurses and a sample of patients (perhaps representatives of your patient participation group if you have one).
- Gather or retrieve data on the number of laboratory and imaging tests undertaken in one month, the methods used for transmitting the results to patients and an estimate of the time and costs involved.
- Estimate the costs of setting up a new system whereby patients leave their mobile number when the tests are arranged and a nurse or suitably trained secretary or receptionist texts the patient when the results arrive.
- Try the new system for a month and record any problems, technical or interpersonal. Discuss the outcome with the practice team and patient representatives.
- Ask parents and carers of pre-school children to inform the practice of their mobile telephone numbers as they attend for appointments or when they are visited, for example by the child and family nurse. Investigate the costs and benefits of installing a software program that sends text messages to remind parents and carers of upcoming vaccinations and developmental checks:

www.textmagic.co.uk/
www.csoft.co.uk/
www.fastsms.co.uk/
www.ccl.co.uk/text_messaging.html [all accessed November 2006].

Exercise 20

Consider investing in a digital camera for the practice. After obtaining informed consent, use it to photograph patients' rashes and skin lesions when you are unsure of the diagnosis. Show the images to a colleague for second opinion. If your local dermatologist in amenable, ask him or her if you can email the image instead of making a referral. Patients must be aware that information about them is being transmitted in this way, since email attachments are not secure and can be saved, copied and forwarded to third parties without the knowledge of patient or clinician.

References

1. CEC DG XIII. *Research and Technology Development on Telematics Systems in Health Care*. Annual technical report on RTD in heath care. Brussels: AIM, 1993.
2. Mair F and Whitten P. Systematic review of studies of patient satisfaction with telemedicine. *British Medical Journal* 2000;**320**:1517–20.
3. Conrath D, Buckingham P, Dunn E and Swanson N. An experimental evaluation of alternative communication systems as used for medical diagnosis. *Behavioral Science* 1975;**20**:296–305.
4. Itzhak B, Weinberger T, Berkovitch E and Reis S. Telemedicine in primary care in Israel. *Journal of Telemedicine and Telecare* 1998;**4**:11–14.
5. Malone F, Callaghan C, Chan D, Sheets S and Person D. Caring for children with asthma through teleconsultation: 'ECHO-Pac, the electronic children's hospital of the Pacific'. *Telemedicine Journal and e-Health* 2004;**10**:138–46.
6. Whitten PS, Mair FS, Haycox A, May CR, Williams TL and Hellmich S. Systematic review of cost effectiveness studies of telemedicine interventions. *British Medical Journal* 2002;**324**:1434–7.
7. Whittaker S, Adkins S, Phillips R, Jones J, Horsley M and Kelley G. Success factors in the long-term sustainability of a telediabetes programme. *Journal of Telemedicine and Telecare* 2004;**10**:84–8.
8. Norris T, Hart G, Larson E, Tarczy-Hornoch P, Masuda D, Fuller S, *et al*. Low-bandwidth, low-cost telemedicine consultations in rural family practice. *Journal of the American Board of Family Practice* 2002;**15**:123–7.
9. Wallace P, Haines A, Harrison R, Barber J, Thompson S, Jacklin P, *et al*. Joint teleconsultations (virtual outreach) versus standard outpatient appointments for patients referred by their general practitioner for a specialist opinion: a randomised trial. *The Lancet* 2002;**359**:1961–8.
10. Jacklin PB, Roberts JA, Wallace P, Haines A, Harrison R, Barber JA, *et al*. Virtual outreach: economic evaluation of joint teleconsultations for patients referred by their general practitioner for a specialist opinion. *British Medical Journal* 2003;**327**:84.
11. Baldwin L, Clarke M, Hands L, Knott M and Jones R. The effect of telemedicine on consultation time. *Journal of Telemedicine and Telecare* 2003;**9**:71–3.
12. Eisenberg M, Hallstrom A, Carter B, Cummins R, Bergner L and Pierce J. Emergency CPR instruction via telephone. *American Journal of Public Health* 1985;**75**:47–50.
13. Molinari G, Reboa G, Frascio M, Leoncini M, Rolandi A, Balzan C, *et al*. The role of telecardiology in supporting the decision-making process of general practitioners during the management of patients with suspected cardiac events. *Journal of Telemedicine and Telecare* 2002;**8**:97–101.
14. Scalvini S, Zanelli E, Conti C, Volterrani M, Pollina R, Giordano A, *et al*. Assessment of prehospital chest pain using telecardiology. *Journal of Telemedicine and Telecare* 2002;**8**:231–6.
15. Zenk B, Bratton R, Flipse T and Page E. Accuracy of detecting irregular cardiac rhythms via telemedicine. *Journal of Telemedicine and Telecare* 2004;**10**:55–8.
16. Gilmour E, Campbell S, Loane M, Esmail A, Griffiths C, Roland M, *et al*. Comparison of teleconsultations and face-to-face consultations: preliminary results of a United Kingdom multicentre teledermatology study. *British Journal of Dermatology* 1998;**139**:81–7.
17. Eedy D and Wootton R. Teledermatology: a review. *British Journal of Dermatology* 2001;**144**:696–707.
18. Lawton S, English J, McWilliam J, Wildgust L and Patel R. Development of a district-wide teledermatology service. *Nursing Times* 2004;**100**:38–41.
19. Collins K, Walters S and Bowns I. Patient satisfaction with teledermatology: quantitative and qualitative results from a randomized controlled trial. *Journal of Telemedicine and Telecare* 2004;**10**:29–33.
20. Collins K, Bowns I and Walters S. General practitioners' perceptions of asynchronous telemedicine in a randomized controlled trial of teledermatology. *Journal of Telemedicine and Telecare* 2004;**10**:94–8.
21. Etherington IJ. Telecolposcopy – a feasibility study in primary care. *Journal of Telemedicine and Telecare* 2002;**8**:22–4.

22. Etherington IJ, Watts A, Hughes E and Lester H. The use of telemedicine in primary care for women with cervical cytological abnormalities. *Journal of Telemedicine and Telecare* 2002;**8**:17–19.
23. Wittson C, Affleck D and Johnson V. Two-way television in group therapy. *Mental Hospitals* 1961;**2**:22–3.
24. Evans M, Kessler D, Lewis G, Peters T and Sharp D. Assessing mental health in primary care research using standardized scales: can it be carried out over the telephone? *Psychological Medicine* 2004;**34**:157–62.
25. Hilty D, Luo J, Morache C, Marcelo D and Nesbitt T. Telepsychiatry: an overview for psychiatrists. *CNS Drugs* 2002;**16**:527–48.
26. McLaren P, Ahlbom J, Riley A, Mohammedali A and Denis M. The North Lewisham telepsychiatry project: beyond the pilot phase. *Journal of Telemedicine and Telecare* 2002;**8**:98–100.
27. The Audit Commission. *Assistive Technology: Independence and Wellbeing 4*. www.audit-commission.gov.uk/reports/NATIONAL-REPORT.asp?CategoryID=&ProdID=BB070AC2-A23A-4478-BD69-4C19BE942722 [accessed November 2006]. 2004.
28. Kobb R, Hoffman N, Lodge R and Kline S. Enhancing elder chronic care through technology and care coordination: report from a pilot. *Telemedicine Journal and e-Health* 2003;**9**:189–95.
29. Department of Health. *Long Term Conditions National Service Framework*. www.dh.gov.uk/PolicyAndGuidance/HealthAndSocialCareTopics/LongTermConditions/fs/en [accessed November 2006]. 2004.
30. Neal R, Pascoe S and Allgar V. Alternative forms of consulting: survey of patients and GPs about their consultations. *Family Practice* 2004;**21**:140–2.
31. Stevenson M, Marsh J and Roderick E. Can patients predict which consultations can be dealt with by telephone? *British Journal of General Practice* 1998;**48**:1772.
32. Moyer C, Stern D, Dobias K, Cox D and Katz S. Bridging the electronic divide: patient and provider perspectives on e-mail communication in primary care. *American Journal of Managed Care* 2002;**8**:427–33.
33. Skolnick A. Experts explore emerging information technologies' effects on medicine. *Journal of the American Medical Association* 1996;**275**:669–70.
34. Peters R and Sikorski R. Digital dialogue: sharing information and interests on the Internet. *Journal of the American Medical Association* 1997;**277**:1258–60.
35. Green L. A better way to keep in touch with patients: electronic mail. *Medical Economics* 1996;**73**:153.
36. Neville R. E-mail consultations in general practice (letter). *British Journal of General Practice* 2004;**54**:546.
37. Houston T, Sands D, Nash B and Ford D. Experiences of physicians who frequently use e-mail with patients. *Health Communication* 2003;**15**:515–25.
38. Spielberg A. On call and online: sociohistorical, legal and ethical implications of e-mail for the patient–physician relationship. *Journal of the American Medical Association* 1998;**280**:1353–9.
39. Eminovic N, Wyatt J, Tarpey A, Murray G and Ingrams G. First evaluation of the NHS direct online clinical enquiry service: a nurse-led web chat triage service for the public. *Journal of Medical Internet Research* 2004;**6**:e17.
40. Kobak K, Taylor L, Dottl S, Greist J, Jefferson J, Burroughs D, *et al*. A computer-administered telephone interview to identify mental disorders. *Journal of the American Medical Association* 1997;**278**:905–10.
41. Stuart G, Laraia M, Ornstein S and Nietert P. An interactive voice response system to enhance antidepressant medication compliance. *Topics in Health Information Management* 2003;**24**:15–20.
42. Pal B. The doctor will text you now: is there a role for the mobile telephone in health care? (personal view). *British Medical Journal* 2003;**326**:607.
43. Neville R, Greene A, McLeod J, Tracy A and Surie J. Mobile phone text messaging can help young people manage asthma (letter). *British Medical Journal* 2002;**325**:600.

Summary

This book has covered a range of telephone communication and consultation issues:

- factors that modify verbal and non-verbal communication in the absence of visual and other sensory cues, and how these affect the diagnostic accuracy and decision-making behaviour of health professionals
- educational interventions and patient-centred telephone consultation models that attempt to compensate for the relatively cueless environment of the telephone
- guidance on how to assess and manage common clinical problems presenting by telephone in the context of uncertainty
- the multi-disciplinary and inter-professional nature of telephone medicine, and other methods of conducting consultations at a distance.

The aim of this summary is to synthesise these issues and enable the reader to embark on telephone-based medicine with greater confidence and self-awareness, and with a repertoire of skills to respond to the demands of contemporary primary care. It closes with the patients' perspective since the people for whom health services exist also need to feel confident and skilled in telephone communication with practitioners.

Consultation skills

Several consultation tasks and stages were identified from the literature in Chapter 2:

1. identify oneself and caller, the latter being the patient whenever possible
2. gather information from the caller's initial message, the social context and the clinical history
3. address both the biomedical aspects of the problem as well as the patient's perspective
4. give a diagnosis or interpretation of the patient's problem with an explanation or a summary
5. signpost the point at which a triage or management decision must be made
6. negotiate the outcome according to agreed guidelines
7. make follow-up arrangements and provide a safety net
8. prepare for the next call and be professionally safe, with good record-keeping of particular importance.

Each of these tasks and stages requires communication skills as well as the application of clinical knowledge, the one for enabling the patient or carer to express their problem as fully and accurately as possible, the other to determine the diagnosis and options for management. Knowledge can be communicated to the caller in the form of explanation or advice, and communication skills can facilitate the negotiation process involved in collaborative decision-making. The interdependent and intertwined nature of process and content in the consultation has been summarised elsewhere.[1]

Identification

Formal introduction and mutual identification help to set the professional tone of the consultation and avoids either party making assumptions. It is not only the clinician who is without the usual visual cues to help in the communication and management processes; the caller may also need help to adopt the appropriate socially and institutionally determined role of 'patient' in his or her home or work environment. The opening statements of the doctor or nurse, their content, style and non-verbal features, will determine how well and how much the patient communicates in the subsequent narrative. The patient needs to have answers to the following initial concerns:

- will the doctor/nurse be too busy to deal with my problem?
- will he or she think my problem is too minor to worry about?
- will he or she understand that I'm trying to save time by consulting in this way?

Information-gathering

Information is collected through multiple channels and assimilated into a meaningful whole in the clinician's mind's eye. Triage nurses explain how they visualise their telephone patients and this process can extend beyond the patient's physical and mental state to his or her environment. Content needed to clarify the picture such as the appearance of a rash, how many antidepressant tablets are left in the packet or the rate and rhythm of the heart may be acquired by asking the patient or carer to become an extension of the health professional's eyes and hands. The biopsychosocial nature of many primary care presentations requires the clinician to address the disease and associated ideas, concerns, expectations and effects on life and livelihood. Empathy is easier to express in the face-to-face consultation because the clinician can use posture, facial expressions and touch as well as make empathic statements. Telephone empathy not only requires the projection of oneself down the cable to the patient's side to share in the illness experience but also restricts the GP to verbal empathic statements.

Decision-making and accuracy

Studies of decision-making by doctors and nurses in telephone consultations outlined in Chapters 3 and 6 identified features that reflect different clinical reasoning processes. The more experienced clinicians elicit minimal information from callers and are quick to make management decisions and spend more time explaining and advising. Novices ask more questions before reaching a diagnosis through long-winded hypothesis generating and testing, and are relatively weak on explanation and advice. These decision-making styles both have their strengths and weakness. The expert draws from experience and recognises the 'pattern' of an illness presentation. His or her level of uncertainty is determined by the clarity of the clinical picture obtained through the history and by the knowledge of disease prevalence in the population. The novice has not yet built up a collection of presentations and uncertainty is high. Anxiety about missing significant disease leads to a greater consumption of healthcare resources. The telephone consultation as a 'test' when applied by the expert performs with high specificity: this doctor or nurse will correctly advise patients with self-limiting problems to manage their symptoms with home remedies the vast majority of the time. The novice's consultations will be more sensitive because the threshold for arranging a face-to-face consultation will be lower, reducing the risk of missing an important diagnosis, but less specific because of the 'false positives' he or she is likely to generate.

Another important factor in diagnostic accuracy relates to the 'mind snapping shut' phenomenon described in Chapter 3. Electing not to share thinking with a patient and denying him or her the opportunity to express additional concerns or mention other problems leads to narrow biomedical diagnoses[2] and unilateral doctor-centred treatment plans.[3] Clinicians aware of this premature decision-making feature of telephone consultations can compensate by deliberately signposting the point at which they feel ready to make a decision but allow the patient to intervene with ideas if the complete picture of the predicament has not yet been described.

Negotiation

Negotiation is less stressful when the clinician has a full account of the patient's predicament and when the patient feels that he or she has been listened to. Conditions that are amenable to treatment by protocol – either adopted from national guidance or developed at practice level – should empower the clinician to offer standard treatment and advice.

Safety-netting

Ending a telephone consultation should include shared thoughts on 'what ifs', such as what if things get worse, what if the treatment fails and what if the diagnosis is wrong. It seems that the more opportunity a patient is given to make further contact the less he or she will actually call again.[4]

Keeping good records

Time can be saved during telephone consultations by making notes during the conversation, a practice usually frowned upon in the face-to-face interview. The use of hands-free telephone facilities enables the doctor or nurse to type information into an electronic medical record as it is elicited, just as nurses using decision-support software do in order to help them in their lines of questioning and management of the patient.

Facilitating teamwork

The GP's role in primary care has evolved to include the coordination of the many community-based health professionals involved in patient care. Nurses, midwives, physiotherapists and pharmacists are now autonomous individuals with their own caseloads, and GP expertise is part of the primary care 'skill mix'. Team-working is vital in order to fulfil the requirements of the General Medical Services contract, especially in areas such as access, chronic disease management and health promotion. David Haslam, current President of the RCGP, has set out the contemporary role of the GP in the NHS as a whole, emphasising the trust-worthiness, breadth of skills, depth of understanding and interpretation of patients' problems and flexibility of family doctors, as well as their ability to contain health service costs through appropriate gate-keeping.[5]

Whether through triage or open-access appointment systems, patients are able to present any given problem to a range of clinicians in primary care. In order to avoid inconsistent treatment and advice on the part of the clinical team, and ensure appropriate navigation of the system on the part of the patient, it is important that policies and boundaries are discussed and agreed upon within the primary health team. This requires protected time for personal and team development, review of current evidence and contractual obligations, and the participation and co-agreement of patients through local patient participation groups. Individual practice teams can reach a consensus on what proportion of clinical time should be set aside for telephone consultations, what acute and chronic conditions are to be managed this way, the specific advice to be given for each condition through practice protocols and the balance of patient- and practice-initiated calls. Such a consistent and concerted approach to patient care will help not only the relationship between the practice and its patient population but also the efficiency with which the practice carries out its duties.

Teamwork involves cooperating with colleagues in secondary care through patient referral, admission and continuing community care following discharge. The GP is usually in a position to judge whether a referral is likely to benefit a patient but uncertainty about the appropriateness of a referral can be reduced by a preliminary telephone call to the relevant consultant or junior colleague. Some referrals can be avoided or given higher priority through initial telephone contact as it can be difficult to convey the nuances of a case through a referral letter. GPs appreciate being forewarned about certain hospital discharges so that they can prepare the team for home visits and family support, particularly in palliative care. Such advice may come via a brief telephone message accompanied by a faxed summary.

The patients' perspective

To make the most of a telephone consultation, patients and carers need a reasonable amount of lay medical knowledge but also need to be aware of their own interpersonal and communication skills. Patients not only have symptoms but those symptoms also exist in a context that includes psychosocial factors and previous experience of illness and of contact with health professionals.[6] Anxiety about a health problem may impair communication, either by reducing the amount of information taken in from a doctor giving advice or by compounding the severity of the true situation with emotive words or other embellishment. Zola[7] described triggers that make people decide to consult about a symptom and the factors involved in crossing their consulting threshold.

Organisations that support patients in their use of NHS services such as the charity Developing Patient Partnerships (www.dpp.org.uk/ [accessed November 2006]) produce written guidance:

• *Where to Go When You are Unwell*[8]
• *Caring for Kids: A self-care guide to childhood ailments*.[9]

For a comprehensive source of information NHS Direct can be contacted by telephone (0845 46 47 in England and Wales; 08454 24 24 24 in Scotland) or via the internet (www.nhsdirect.nhs.uk/ [accessed November 2006]).

References

1. Kurtz S, Silverman D, Benson J and Draper J. Marrying content and process in clinical method teaching: enhancing the Calgary–Cambridge guides. *Academic Medicine* 2003;**78**:802–9.
2. East Anglia Communications Skills Cascade Facilitators. *Are There Problems in Communication between Doctors and Patients?* www.skillscascade.com/files/commresearch.htm [accessed November 2006]. 2002.
3. Tuckett D, Boulton M, Olson C and Williams A. *Meetings between Experts*. London: Tavistock, 1985.
4. Curtis P and Evens S. The telephone interview. In: Lipkin M, Putman S, Lazare A, eds. *The Medical Interview*. New York: Springer-Verlag, 1995, pp. 187–95.
5. Haslam D. *The Future of General Practice: A Statement by the Royal College of General Practitioners*. www.rcgp.org.uk/PDF/Corp_future_of_general_practice.pdf [accessed November 2006]. 2004.
6. Hopton J, Hogg R and McKee I. Patients' accounts of calling the doctor out of hours: qualitative study in one general practice. *British Medical Journal* 1996;**313**:991–4.
7. Zola IK. Pathways to the doctor – from person to patient. *Social Science Medicine* 1973;**7**:677–89.
8. Developing Patient Partnerships. *Where to Go When You are Unwell*. www.dpp.org.uk/en/1/camuos.qxml [accessed November 2006]. 2004.
9. Developing Patient Partnerships. *Caring for Kids: A self-care guide to childhood ailments*. www.dpp.org.uk/en/1/camcfk.qxml [accessed November 2006]. 2003.

Index